Holistic Health

A Comprehensive Guide to Mind-Body Wellness

Park Windsor

Contents

Chapter 1
Introduction to Holistic Health

Defining Holistic Health

Holistic health, also known as holistic healing or holistic wellness, is an approach to healthcare that emphasizes the interconnectedness of the mind, body, and spirit in achieving overall well-being. At its core, holistic health recognizes that each individual is a complex system comprised of various dimensions, including physical, mental, emotional, social, and spiritual aspects, all of which play vital roles in determining one's health and vitality.

Rather than focusing solely on treating symptoms or isolated health issues, holistic health seeks to address the underlying root causes of illness or imbalance by considering the whole person and their unique circumstances. This approach encompasses a wide range of modalities and practices, including conventional medicine, alternative therapies, lifestyle interventions, and self-care strategies, with the goal of promoting optimal health and preventing disease.

Key principles of holistic health include:

1. **Wholeness:** Recognizing that individuals are integrated beings with interconnected physical, mental, emotional, and spiritual dimensions.

2. **Prevention:** Emphasizing proactive measures to maintain health and wellness, rather than solely reacting to illness or symptoms.

3. **Individuality:** Acknowledging that each person has unique needs, preferences, and circumstances that influence their health journey.

4. **Empowerment:** Encouraging individuals to take an active role in their own health and well-being through informed decision-making and self-care practices.

5. **Balance:** Striving for equilibrium and harmony among the various aspects of life, including work, relationships, leisure, and self-care.

6. **Integration:** Integrating conventional and complementary approaches to healthcare in a cohesive and personalized manner.

The Interconnectedness of Mind, Body, and Spirit

The interconnectedness of mind, body, and spirit is a fundamental concept in holistic health, highlighting the dynamic relationship between these three aspects of human existence.

1. **Mind:** The mind encompasses cognitive functions, emotions, thoughts, beliefs, and perceptions. It influences our behaviors, decisions, and experiences. Mental health is closely tied to physical health, as stress, anxiety, and other psychological factors can impact bodily functions and overall well-being. Practices such as mindfulness meditation, cognitive-behavioral therapy, and positive affirmations are used to cultivate mental wellness and promote harmony within the mind-body-spirit connection.

2. **Body:** The body refers to the physical vessel through which we experience the world. Physical health involves the proper functioning of bodily systems, organs, tissues, and cells. The body's health is influenced by lifestyle factors such as diet, exercise, sleep, and environmental exposures. Holistic health recognizes that the body's physical state can affect mental and emotional well-being, and vice versa. For example, chronic stress can manifest as physical symptoms like muscle tension, headaches, or digestive issues. Holistic practices such as yoga, acupuncture, massage therapy, and nutritional therapy aim to optimize physical health and restore balance to the body-mind-spirit connection.

3. **Spirit:** The spirit encompasses one's inner essence, values, beliefs, and sense of purpose or connection to something greater than oneself. It is often associated with concepts of meaning, transcendence, and existential fulfillment. Spiritual health involves nurturing a sense of wholeness, meaning, and connection in life. For some, this may involve religious or spiritual practices, while for others, it may involve activities such as spending time in nature, practicing gratitude, or engaging in creative expression. Cultivating spiritual well-being can enhance overall resilience, coping skills, and quality of life.

In holistic health philosophy, the mind, body, and spirit are viewed as interconnected and inseparable aspects of human experience. Imbalances or disturbances in one aspect can impact the others, leading to symptoms of dis-ease or discomfort. Therefore, holistic healing approaches seek to address the root causes of imbalance by considering the interconnectedness of these dimensions and promoting holistic well-being across mind, body, and spirit. By nurturing harmony and alignment within the mind-body-spirit connection, individuals can experience greater vitality, resilience, and fulfillment in their lives.

Historical Perspectives on Holistic Healing

Historical perspectives on holistic healing trace back to ancient civilizations where various cultures embraced the interconnectedness of mind, body, and spirit in maintaining health and well-being. Here are some key historical perspectives on holistic healing:

1. **Ancient Traditions:** Many ancient cultures, including those of China, India, Greece, and Egypt, developed holistic healing systems based on the concept of balance and harmony within the body and with nature. Traditional Chinese Medicine (TCM) emphasizes the flow of vital energy (Qi) through meridians in the body, with practices such as acupuncture, herbal medicine, tai chi, and qigong aimed at restoring balance. Similarly, Ayurveda, the ancient healing system of India, focuses on individual constitution (doshas) and employs herbal remedies, dietary adjustments, yoga, and meditation to promote holistic wellness.

2. **Greek Medicine:** In ancient Greece, the physician Hippocrates laid the foundation for Western holistic healing with his holistic approach to medicine. He emphasized the importance of diet, exercise, rest, and emotional well-being in maintaining health, famously stating, "Let food be thy medicine and medicine be thy food." Hippocratic medicine focused on treating the whole person rather than just symptoms and recognized the interconnectedness of bodily systems.

3. **Medieval Healing Practices:** During the Middle Ages, holistic healing traditions persisted alongside emerging scientific and religious paradigms. Herbalism, naturopathy, and folk medicine thrived, with

healers incorporating spiritual and energetic elements into their practices. Monastic gardens cultivated medicinal herbs, and holistic healing methods were often intertwined with religious rituals and beliefs.

4. **Renaissance and Enlightenment:** The Renaissance and Enlightenment periods in Europe saw a resurgence of interest in holistic healing as scholars revisited ancient texts and embraced empirical observation and experimentation.

5. **Modern Holistic Health Movement:** The 19th and 20th centuries witnessed the development of modern holistic health movements in response to the limitations of conventional medicine and the growing interest in alternative healing modalities.

Throughout history, holistic healing has evolved in response to cultural, social, and scientific developments, yet its underlying principles of interconnectedness, balance, and individualized care remain central to promoting health and well-being across mind, body, and spirit. Today, holistic approaches to health continue to gain recognition and acceptance, complementing conventional medical practices and offering comprehensive strategies for achieving optimal wellness.

The Role of Holistic Health in Modern Wellness

In the modern era, holistic health plays a crucial role in promoting comprehensive wellness by addressing the interconnectedness of mind, body, and spirit. Here's how holistic health contributes to modern wellness:

1. **Comprehensive Approach:** Holistic health considers the entirety of an individual's well-being, recognizing that optimal health extends beyond physical symptoms to encompass mental, emotional, social, and spiritual aspects. This comprehensive approach allows for a deeper understanding of the root causes of imbalance and offers personalized strategies for promoting overall wellness.

2. **Preventive Care:** Holistic health emphasizes preventive care and lifestyle interventions aimed at maintaining health and preventing illness. By addressing underlying imbalances and risk factors, holistic approaches help individuals reduce their susceptibility to chronic diseases and enhance their resilience to stressors, thus promoting long-term wellness and vitality.

3. **Integration of Modalities:** Holistic health integrates a diverse range of healing modalities, including conventional medicine, alternative therapies, mind-body practices, nutritional interventions, and self-care techniques. This integrative approach acknowledges the value of combining different treatment options to address the complex needs of individuals and optimize health outcomes.

4. **Empowerment and Self-Care:** Holistic health empowers individuals to take an active role in their own health and well-being. Through education, self-awareness, and self-care practices, individuals learn to make informed choices that support their holistic wellness journey. By cultivating a sense of agency and autonomy, holistic approaches foster greater resilience and self-efficacy in managing health challenges.

5. **Personalized and Patient-Centered Care:** Holistic health emphasizes personalized, patient-centered care that considers each individual's unique needs, preferences, and circumstances. Practitioners take the time to listen to patients' concerns, understand their health goals, and collaborate with them to develop tailored treatment plans that address their holistic wellness needs. This approach fosters trust, communication, and mutual respect in the therapeutic relationship.

6. **Promotion of Mental and Emotional Well-Being:** Holistic health recognizes the profound influence of mental and emotional factors on overall health and wellness. Mind-body practices such as meditation, yoga, mindfulness, and breathwork are integral components of holistic approaches, promoting relaxation, stress reduction, emotional balance, and mental clarity. By nurturing mental and emotional well-being, holistic health contributes to resilience, coping skills, and quality of life.

Integrating Holistic Principles into Everyday Life

Integrating holistic principles into everyday life is essential for promoting mind-body wellness and achieving optimal health and vitality. Here are some practical ways to incorporate holistic health practices into your daily routine:

1. **Mindfulness Meditation:** Set aside time each day for mindfulness meditation to cultivate present-moment awareness, reduce stress, and promote mental clarity. Start with just a few minutes of focused breathing or body scan meditation and gradually increase the duration as you build your practice.

2. **Nutrient-Dense Diet:** Focus on consuming whole, nutrient-dense foods such as fruits, vegetables, whole grains, lean proteins, and healthy fats. Aim for a balanced diet that provides essential vitamins, minerals, antioxidants, and phytonutrients to support overall health and vitality.

3. **Regular Exercise:** Engage in regular physical activity that incorporates both aerobic exercise and strength training. Find activities that you enjoy, whether it's walking, jogging, cycling, yoga, or dancing, and make movement a regular part of your daily routine to improve cardiovascular health, muscle strength, flexibility, and mood.

4. **Stress Management Techniques:** Practice stress management techniques such as deep breathing exercises, progressive muscle relaxation, guided imagery, or journaling to reduce stress levels and promote relaxation. Incorporate stress-relieving activities into your daily routine, such as taking short breaks to go for a walk, spending time in nature, or listening to calming music.

5. **Quality Sleep:** Prioritize getting adequate and restful sleep each night by establishing a regular sleep schedule, creating a relaxing bedtime routine, and optimizing your sleep environment. Aim for 7-9 hours of quality sleep to support physical, mental, and emotional well-being.

6. **Mindful Eating:** Practice mindful eating by paying attention to your body's hunger and fullness cues, savoring each bite, and eating slowly and attentively. Avoid distractions such as screens or multitasking while eating, and choose nourishing foods that support your health goals.

7. **Cultivating Relationships:** Nurture meaningful relationships with friends, family, and community members by prioritizing quality time together, expressing gratitude and appreciation, and offering support and empathy. Social connections are essential for emotional well-being and provide a sense of belonging and connection.

8. **Self-Care Practices:** Incorporate self-care practices into your daily routine to nurture your physical, mental, and emotional well-being. This may include activities such as taking relaxing baths, practicing self-massage, indulging in hobbies or creative pursuits, or simply taking time for yourself to rest and recharge.

9. **Connecting with Nature:** Spend time outdoors and connect with nature to promote grounding, stress reduction, and overall well-being. Take walks in the park, go hiking or camping, garden, or simply sit outside and soak up the natural beauty around you.

10. **Spiritual Exploration:** Explore practices that nourish your spiritual well-being and foster a sense of connection to something greater than yourself. This may involve meditation, prayer, mindfulness, attending religious or spiritual services, or engaging in activities that align with your personal beliefs and values.

Chapter 2
Holistic Nutrition

Understanding the Role of Nutrition in Holistic Health

Understanding the role of nutrition in holistic health is essential for promoting overall well-being and achieving mind-body wellness. Nutrition is not just about fueling the body; it also influences mental, emotional, and spiritual aspects of health. Here's how nutrition plays a vital role in holistic health:

1. **Nourishment for the Body:** Nutrition provides essential nutrients, including carbohydrates, proteins, fats, vitamins, minerals, and water, that are necessary for the proper functioning of bodily systems and processes. A well-balanced diet supports physical health by promoting optimal organ function, cellular repair and regeneration, immune system strength, and energy production.

2. **Supporting Mental Health:** Nutrition plays a significant role in mental health and cognitive function. Certain nutrients, such as omega-3 fatty acids, B vitamins, and antioxidants, support brain health and may help reduce the risk of mental health conditions such as depression, anxiety, and cognitive decline. Conversely, poor nutrition, including diets high in processed foods, sugar, and unhealthy fats, has been linked to an increased risk of mental health disorders.

3. **Emotional Well-Being:** Nutrition can impact emotional well-being by influencing mood, stress levels, and emotional resilience. Consuming nutrient-dense foods that support stable blood sugar levels and provide essential nutrients can help regulate mood and reduce the risk of mood swings, irritability, and emotional instability. Additionally, certain foods, such as those rich in tryptophan (an amino acid precursor to serotonin), may have mood-enhancing effects.

4. **Gut Health and Immunity:** The gut microbiome, which consists of trillions of bacteria residing in the digestive tract, plays a crucial role in immune function, digestion, nutrient absorption, and overall health. Nutrition plays a key role in shaping the composition and diversity of the gut microbiome, with dietary factors such as fiber, prebiotics, probiotics, and fermented foods supporting a healthy gut ecosystem. A

balanced diet that promotes gut health can enhance immune function and reduce the risk of chronic diseases.

5. **Spiritual and Energetic Nutrition:** In holistic health, nutrition is also viewed from a spiritual and energetic perspective, recognizing that food carries not only physical nutrients but also energetic qualities that can influence one's spiritual well-being. Some holistic healing traditions emphasize the importance of consuming whole, unprocessed foods that are energetically vibrant and align with one's personal constitution and spiritual beliefs. Mindful eating practices, gratitude rituals, and conscious food preparation are ways to infuse spiritual intention into nutrition.

6. **Individualized Approach:** Holistic nutrition takes into account individual differences, preferences, and needs, recognizing that there is no one-size-fits-all approach to diet and nutrition. Personalized nutrition considers factors such as genetics, biochemistry, lifestyle, cultural background, food sensitivities, and health goals to develop tailored dietary recommendations that support optimal health and well-being.

Whole Foods and Nutrient-Dense Eating

Whole foods and nutrient-dense eating are foundational principles of holistic nutrition, emphasizing the importance of consuming foods in their natural, unprocessed state to support optimal health and wellness. Here's a closer look at the significance of whole foods and nutrient-dense eating in holistic health:

1. **Nutrient Density:** Nutrient-dense foods are rich in essential nutrients such as vitamins, minerals, antioxidants, and phytonutrients relative to their calorie content. These foods provide the body with a wide array of nutrients necessary for optimal functioning and overall well-being. Examples of nutrient-dense foods include fruits, vegetables, whole grains, legumes, nuts, seeds, lean proteins, and healthy fats.

2. **Minimally Processed:** Whole foods are minimally processed or refined and retain their natural nutrient content, fiber, and beneficial phytochemicals. Unlike processed foods, which often contain added sugars, unhealthy fats, sodium, and artificial ingredients, whole foods offer superior nutritional value and support various aspects of health, including digestion, metabolism, immune function, and heart health.

3. **Fiber-Rich:** Whole foods are typically high in dietary fiber, which plays a crucial role in digestive health, blood sugar regulation, cholesterol management, and weight management. Fiber promotes satiety, helps maintain healthy bowel movements, and supports the growth of beneficial gut bacteria. Whole plant foods such as fruits, vegetables, whole grains, legumes, and nuts are excellent sources of dietary fiber.

4. **Balanced Macronutrients:** Whole foods provide a balanced mix of macronutrients—carbohydrates, proteins, and fats—that are essential for energy production, tissue repair, hormone synthesis, and other physiological functions. By incorporating a variety of whole foods into your diet, you can ensure adequate intake of all macronutrients and support overall health and vitality.

5. **Phytonutrients and Antioxidants:** Whole foods are rich in phytonutrients and antioxidants, bioactive compounds that have protective effects against oxidative stress, inflammation, and chronic diseases. Phytonutrients and antioxidants contribute to the vibrant colors, flavors, and aromas of plant foods and offer numerous health benefits, including immune support, anti-inflammatory effects, and enhanced cellular repair and regeneration.

6. **Environmental and Sustainability Benefits:** Choosing whole foods over processed foods can have positive environmental and sustainability implications. Whole foods often require fewer resources and have a lower environmental footprint compared to heavily processed and packaged foods. By supporting local and sustainable agriculture and minimizing food waste, individuals can contribute to environmental conservation and promote holistic health on a broader scale.

Mindful Eating Practices

Mindful eating practices are integral to holistic nutrition, emphasizing the importance of cultivating awareness, presence, and intentionality around food consumption. By practicing mindful eating, individuals can develop a healthier relationship with food, enhance digestion, and promote overall well-being. Here are some key principles of mindful eating:

1. **Eat with Awareness:** Pay attention to your eating experience by slowing down, savoring each bite, and fully engaging your senses. Notice the colors, textures, aromas, and flavors of your food, and appreciate the nourishment it provides to your body.

2. **Listen to Your Body:** Tune into your body's hunger and fullness cues to guide your eating decisions. Eat when you are hungry and stop when you are comfortably satisfied, rather than eating mindlessly or according to external cues such as emotions or social pressure.

3. **Practice Non-Judgment:** Approach food without judgment or criticism, and cultivate a non-reactive attitude towards your eating habits and preferences. Be curious and compassionate towards yourself, recognizing that every eating experience is an opportunity for learning and growth.

4. **Be Present:** Be present with your food and the act of eating, avoiding distractions such as screens, work, or multitasking. Create a calm and focused eating environment that allows you to fully immerse yourself in the experience of nourishing your body.

5. **Cultivate Gratitude:** Cultivate gratitude for the food you are eating and the people, animals, and ecosystems involved in its production. Take a moment to express gratitude before each meal, acknowledging the abundance and interconnectedness of life.

6. **Practice Mindful Portion Control:** Pay attention to portion sizes and serve yourself appropriate amounts of food based on your hunger and energy needs. Use mindful portion control techniques such as mindful

plate planning, mindful serving sizes, and mindful eating intervals to support balanced and mindful eating habits.

7. **Engage in Conscious Food Choices:** Make conscious food choices that align with your values, preferences, and health goals. Choose whole, minimally processed foods that nourish your body and support holistic health, and be mindful of the environmental and ethical implications of your food choices.

8. **Savor the Experience:** Take the time to savor the eating experience and fully enjoy the pleasure and satisfaction that comes from eating nourishing and delicious food. Cultivate an attitude of gratitude, joy, and appreciation towards your meals, and savor each moment of nourishment and connection.

Holistic Approaches to Special Diets

Holistic approaches to special diets involve considering the interconnectedness of mind, body, and spirit while addressing specific dietary needs or health conditions. These approaches prioritize whole, nutrient-dense foods and aim to support overall well-being while accommodating individual preferences and requirements. Here are some holistic approaches to special diets:

1. **Plant-Based Diet:** A plant-based diet emphasizes whole, minimally processed plant foods such as fruits, vegetables, whole grains, legumes, nuts, and seeds while minimizing or eliminating animal products. This approach aligns with holistic principles by promoting healthful eating patterns that are rich in fiber, antioxidants, vitamins, and minerals, while also supporting environmental sustainability and animal welfare. A plant-based diet has been associated with numerous health benefits, including reduced risk of chronic diseases such as heart disease, diabetes, and certain cancers.

2. **Gluten-Free Diet:** A gluten-free diet eliminates gluten, a protein found in wheat, barley, rye, and their derivatives, and is essential for individuals with celiac disease or gluten sensitivity. Holistic approaches to a gluten-free diet focus on choosing naturally gluten-free whole

grains such as quinoa, brown rice, millet, and buckwheat, as well as incorporating nutrient-dense foods like fruits, vegetables, lean proteins, and healthy fats. It also involves addressing potential nutrient deficiencies and gut health issues commonly associated with gluten-related disorders.

3. **Paleo Diet:** The Paleo diet, also known as the Paleolithic or caveman diet, emphasizes consuming foods that our ancestors would have eaten during the Paleolithic era, such as lean meats, fish, fruits, vegetables, nuts, and seeds, while avoiding processed foods, grains, dairy, and legumes. Holistic approaches to the Paleo diet focus on choosing high-quality, nutrient-dense foods from sustainable and ethical sources, emphasizing whole foods over processed alternatives, and incorporating mindfulness and gratitude practices into meal planning and preparation.

4. **Low-FODMAP Diet:** The low-FODMAP diet is a dietary approach used to manage symptoms of irritable bowel syndrome (IBS) and other gastrointestinal conditions by reducing intake of certain fermentable carbohydrates (FODMAPs) that can trigger digestive symptoms. Holistic approaches to the low-FODMAP diet involve working with a healthcare provider or registered dietitian to identify trigger foods, experiment with reintroducing FODMAP-containing foods, and focus on gut-healing strategies such as consuming gut-friendly foods, managing stress, and incorporating mindfulness practices into mealtime routines.

5. **Ketogenic Diet:** The ketogenic diet is a high-fat, low-carbohydrate eating plan that has gained popularity for its potential benefits in weight loss, blood sugar regulation, and neurological conditions such as epilepsy. Holistic approaches to the ketogenic diet emphasize choosing healthy fats from sources such as avocados, nuts, seeds, coconut oil, and fatty fish, while also incorporating nutrient-dense vegetables, low-glycemic fruits, and quality proteins. It also involves monitoring electrolyte balance, supporting liver and kidney health, and incorporating lifestyle factors such as stress management and physical activity.

6. **Allergy-Friendly Diet:** An allergy-friendly diet involves avoiding specific foods or ingredients that trigger allergic reactions or

intolerances, such as dairy, eggs, soy, peanuts, tree nuts, shellfish, and wheat. Holistic approaches to an allergy-friendly diet focus on choosing whole, minimally processed foods that are free from allergens, while also addressing nutrient deficiencies, supporting immune function, and promoting gut health through probiotic-rich foods, prebiotic fibers, and anti-inflammatory nutrients.

Balancing Macronutrients for Optimal Wellness

Balancing macronutrients—carbohydrates, proteins, and fats—is essential for optimal wellness and holistic nutrition. Each macronutrient plays a unique role in the body and contributes to overall health and vitality. Here's how to balance macronutrients for optimal wellness in a holistic approach to nutrition:

1. **Carbohydrates:** Carbohydrates are the body's primary source of energy and are found in foods such as fruits, vegetables, grains, legumes, and starchy vegetables. Opt for whole, minimally processed carbohydrates that are rich in fiber, vitamins, and minerals, such as whole grains (brown rice, quinoa, oats), fruits, vegetables, and legumes. These complex carbohydrates provide sustained energy, promote satiety, support digestive health, and help regulate blood sugar levels.

2. **Proteins:** Proteins are essential for building and repairing tissues, synthesizing hormones and enzymes, and supporting immune function. Include a variety of high-quality protein sources in your diet, such as lean meats, poultry, fish, eggs, dairy products, tofu, tempeh, legumes, nuts, and seeds. Aim to distribute protein intake evenly throughout the day to support muscle protein synthesis and maintain satiety. Choose lean proteins and plant-based protein sources whenever possible and opt for organic, grass-fed, or wild-caught options when available.

3. **Fats:** Fats are necessary for hormone production, brain function, cellular integrity, and absorption of fat-soluble vitamins (A, D, E, K). Focus on incorporating healthy fats into your diet, such as monounsaturated fats (olive oil, avocados, nuts, seeds), polyunsaturated fats (fatty fish, flaxseeds, walnuts, chia seeds), and

small amounts of saturated fats (coconut oil, grass-fed butter). Limit intake of trans fats and processed fats found in fried foods, baked goods, and processed snacks. Aim to include a variety of fats in your diet to support overall health and well-being.

4. **Balanced Meals and Snacks:** Aim to create balanced meals and snacks that include a combination of carbohydrates, proteins, and fats to provide sustained energy and satiety. For example, pair whole grains or starchy vegetables with lean protein and healthy fats, such as oatmeal topped with nuts and fruit, a salad with grilled chicken and avocado, or whole grain toast with almond butter and banana. Incorporate a mix of colors, textures, and flavors to make meals more satisfying and enjoyable.

5. **Portion Control and Moderation:** Practice portion control and moderation when it comes to macronutrient intake to ensure balance and prevent overconsumption of any one nutrient. Pay attention to hunger and fullness cues, and aim to eat until you are comfortably satisfied rather than overly full. Be mindful of portion sizes and serving sizes, and avoid oversized portions or excessive calorie intake. Use mindful eating practices to tune into your body's needs and make conscious food choices that support optimal wellness.

6. **Hydration:** In addition to macronutrients, hydration is essential for overall health and well-being. Aim to drink plenty of water throughout the day to stay hydrated and support cellular function, digestion, metabolism, and detoxification. Limit intake of sugary beverages, caffeinated drinks, and alcohol, which can contribute to dehydration and disrupt macronutrient balance.

Chapter 3
Mind–Body Connection

Exploring the Mind-Body Connection

Exploring the mind-body connection reveals the intricate relationship between mental and emotional states and physical health, highlighting the profound impact of thoughts, emotions, beliefs, and attitudes on the body's functioning and well-being. Here are key aspects to consider when delving into the mind-body connection:

1. **Psychoneuroimmunology:** Psychoneuroimmunology is the interdisciplinary field that examines the interactions between psychological processes (such as thoughts, emotions, and behaviors), the nervous system, and the immune system. Research in this field has demonstrated that psychological factors can influence immune function, inflammation, and susceptibility to illness, highlighting the bidirectional relationship between the mind and the body.

2. **Stress Response:** The mind-body connection is particularly evident in the stress response, which involves complex interactions between the brain, endocrine system, autonomic nervous system, and immune system. Chronic stress can dysregulate these systems, leading to heightened inflammation, impaired immune function, and increased risk of chronic diseases such as cardiovascular disease, diabetes, and autoimmune disorders. Mind-body practices such as meditation, yoga, and deep breathing exercises can modulate the stress response and promote relaxation and resilience.

3. **Emotional Health:** Emotions have a profound impact on physical health, with studies linking positive emotions such as joy, gratitude, and optimism to better immune function, cardiovascular health, and longevity, while negative emotions such as anger, fear, and sadness have been associated with increased inflammation, oxidative stress, and disease risk. Cultivating emotional well-being through practices such as mindfulness, self-compassion, and gratitude can support holistic health and enhance resilience to stressors.

4. **Placebo Effect:** The placebo effect illustrates the power of the mind to influence physical health outcomes, even in the absence of active treatment. Placebo responses involve complex neurobiological mechanisms and can lead to improvements in symptoms, pain relief,

and subjective well-being. The placebo effect underscores the importance of psychological factors, such as expectations, beliefs, and perceptions, in shaping health outcomes and highlights the potential for harnessing the mind-body connection in therapeutic interventions.

5. **Mind-Body Therapies:** Mind-body therapies encompass a diverse range of approaches that leverage the mind-body connection to promote health and healing. These therapies include practices such as meditation, yoga, tai chi, qigong, biofeedback, hypnotherapy, guided imagery, and cognitive-behavioral therapy (CBT). Mind-body therapies aim to reduce stress, enhance self-awareness, cultivate emotional resilience, and support holistic well-being by fostering integration and balance between the mind and the body.

6. **Integrative Medicine:** Integrative medicine approaches healthcare with a holistic perspective that recognizes the interconnectedness of mind, body, and spirit. Integrative medicine combines conventional medical treatments with evidence-based complementary therapies, such as acupuncture, chiropractic care, nutritional therapy, and mindfulness-based interventions, to address the physical, psychological, and social dimensions of health. By integrating mind-body approaches into clinical practice, integrative medicine seeks to optimize health outcomes and improve quality of life for individuals with acute and chronic health conditions.

Practices for Mindful Living

Practicing mindful living is an essential aspect of nurturing the mind-body connection and promoting holistic health and wellness. Mindful living involves cultivating present-moment awareness, embracing acceptance and non-judgment, and integrating mindfulness practices into daily life. Here are some practices for mindful living:

1. **Mindful Breathing:** Incorporate mindful breathing exercises into your daily routine to anchor yourself in the present moment and calm the mind. Take a few minutes each day to focus on your breath, noticing the sensations of inhalation and exhalation. You can practice

deep belly breathing, diaphragmatic breathing, or simply observe the natural rhythm of your breath as it flows in and out.

2. **Mindful Eating:** Practice mindful eating by bringing awareness to the sensory experience of eating and savoring each bite of food. Slow down and take the time to notice the colors, textures, aromas, and flavors of your food. Chew slowly and mindfully, paying attention to the taste, texture, and sensations in your mouth. Be present with your meals, and cultivate gratitude for the nourishment they provide to your body.

3. **Body Scan Meditation:** Practice body scan meditation to cultivate awareness of bodily sensations and promote relaxation and self-awareness. Lie down in a comfortable position and bring attention to different parts of your body, starting from the toes and gradually moving up to the head. Notice any areas of tension or discomfort and breathe into them with compassion and acceptance.

4. **Mindful Movement:** Engage in mindful movement practices such as yoga, tai chi, or qigong to connect with your body and cultivate awareness of movement, breath, and energy flow. Pay attention to the sensations in your body as you move through the poses or movements, and practice with a spirit of curiosity, openness, and non-judgment.

5. **Mindful Walking:** Take mindful walks in nature to connect with the present moment and experience the beauty and wonder of the natural world. Focus on each step you take, feeling the ground beneath your feet and the rhythm of your breath. Notice the sights, sounds, and sensations around you, and allow yourself to be fully immersed in the experience of walking.

6. **Gratitude Practice:** Cultivate gratitude by taking time each day to reflect on the things you are grateful for in your life. Keep a gratitude journal and write down three things you are grateful for each day, whether big or small. Express gratitude towards yourself, others, and the world around you, and notice how it shifts your perspective and enhances your sense of well-being.

7. **Mindful Communication:** Practice mindful communication by listening attentively to others with an open heart and mind. Pay

attention to both verbal and non-verbal cues, and communicate with empathy, compassion, and authenticity. Be present with the person you are speaking to, and cultivate deep listening and understanding.

8. **Digital Detox:** Take regular breaks from technology and digital devices to reduce distractions and cultivate presence and mindfulness. Set boundaries around screen time, and engage in activities that nourish your body, mind, and spirit, such as spending time in nature, reading, meditating, or connecting with loved ones face-to-face.

Stress Reduction Techniques

Stress reduction techniques are vital for fostering a balanced mind-body connection and promoting holistic health and wellness. Chronic stress can negatively impact physical, mental, and emotional well-being, making it essential to incorporate effective stress management practices into daily life. Here are some techniques for reducing stress and cultivating a sense of calm and balance:

1. **Mindfulness Meditation:** Mindfulness meditation involves bringing focused attention to the present moment without judgment. Set aside time each day to practice mindfulness meditation, focusing on your breath, bodily sensations, or present-moment experiences. Regular meditation practice can help reduce stress, increase resilience, and cultivate a greater sense of calm and clarity.

2. **Deep Breathing Exercises:** Deep breathing exercises, such as diaphragmatic breathing or belly breathing, can help activate the body's relaxation response and reduce stress levels. Practice deep breathing by inhaling deeply through your nose, allowing your abdomen to expand, and exhaling slowly through your mouth. Repeat this process several times, focusing on the sensations of breathing and the feeling of relaxation spreading throughout your body.

3. **Progressive Muscle Relaxation (PMR):** Progressive muscle relaxation involves systematically tensing and relaxing different muscle groups to release physical tension and promote relaxation. Begin by tensing a specific muscle group for a few seconds, then release the tension and

notice the sensations of relaxation. Move through each muscle group, from your toes to your head, progressively releasing tension and promoting a sense of calm and ease.

4. **Yoga and Tai Chi:** Yoga and Tai Chi are mind-body practices that combine gentle movement, breathwork, and meditation to promote relaxation, flexibility, and stress reduction. Incorporate yoga or Tai Chi into your weekly routine to release tension, improve posture, and cultivate mindfulness and body awareness. Choose gentle, restorative yoga styles or Tai Chi forms that focus on relaxation and stress relief.

5. **Nature Walks and Outdoor Activities:** Spending time in nature can have a calming effect on the mind and body, reducing stress and promoting well-being. Take regular nature walks or engage in outdoor activities such as hiking, gardening, or picnicking to connect with the natural world and experience the benefits of fresh air, sunlight, and green spaces.

6. **Guided Imagery and Visualization:** Guided imagery and visualization techniques involve imagining peaceful and calming scenes or experiences to promote relaxation and stress reduction. Find a quiet, comfortable space to practice guided imagery, listen to guided meditation recordings, or create your own visualization scripts tailored to your preferences and goals.

7. **Mindful Movement Practices:** Engage in mindful movement practices such as walking meditation, qigong, or gentle stretching exercises to promote relaxation and reduce stress. Focus on the sensations of movement, breath, and energy flow, and allow yourself to be fully present in the moment. These practices can help ground you in your body and cultivate a sense of calm and balance.

8. **Self-Care Activities:** Prioritize self-care activities that nourish your body, mind, and spirit and promote relaxation and well-being. Take time each day to engage in activities that bring you joy and rejuvenation, such as reading, listening to music, taking a warm bath, or spending time with loved ones. Set boundaries around work and responsibilities, and make self-care a priority in your daily routine.

The Impact of Thoughts and Emotions on Health

The impact of thoughts and emotions on health is profound, highlighting the intricate connection between mental, emotional, and physical well-being. Here's how thoughts and emotions can influence health in a holistic context:

1. **Stress Response:** Thoughts and emotions play a significant role in the body's stress response. When faced with stressors, whether physical, psychological, or emotional, the brain initiates a cascade of physiological responses, including the release of stress hormones such as cortisol and adrenaline. Chronic stress, fueled by negative thoughts, worry, or unresolved emotions, can dysregulate the stress response system, leading to increased inflammation, immune dysfunction, and a higher risk of stress-related health conditions such as cardiovascular disease, diabetes, and anxiety disorders.

2. **Immune Function:** Thoughts and emotions can modulate immune function, influencing susceptibility to illness and disease. Positive emotions such as joy, gratitude, and optimism have been associated with enhanced immune function, reduced inflammation, and improved resilience to infections. Conversely, negative emotions such as anger, fear, and loneliness have been linked to weakened immune responses and increased vulnerability to illness. The mind-body connection underscores the importance of emotional well-being in supporting immune health and overall resilience.

3. **Psychosomatic Symptoms:** Psychosomatic symptoms are physical manifestations of psychological or emotional distress that have no apparent organic cause. Common examples include headaches, gastrointestinal disturbances, fatigue, and muscle tension. These symptoms arise from the mind-body connection, as the body responds to stress, unresolved emotions, or negative thought patterns with physical symptoms. Addressing underlying psychological or emotional factors through techniques such as cognitive-behavioral therapy (CBT), mindfulness, and stress management can help alleviate psychosomatic symptoms and promote holistic healing.

4. **Mind-Body Medicine:** Mind-body medicine approaches healthcare with a holistic perspective that recognizes the interconnectedness of thoughts, emotions, beliefs, and physical health. Mind-body interventions such as meditation, biofeedback, guided imagery, and relaxation techniques aim to harness the power of the mind to promote healing and well-being. These practices leverage the mind-body connection to reduce stress, enhance self-awareness, and support the body's innate healing mechanisms. Research has shown that mind-body interventions can improve outcomes in various health conditions, including chronic pain, hypertension, insomnia, and mood disorders.

5. **Placebo and Nocebo Effects:** The placebo effect illustrates the power of positive thoughts, beliefs, and expectations to influence health outcomes, even in the absence of active treatment. Conversely, the nocebo effect occurs when negative thoughts or expectations lead to adverse health outcomes or symptoms. Both phenomena highlight the influence of mind-set, perception, and belief systems on health and well-being, underscoring the importance of cultivating positive attitudes and fostering a supportive inner dialogue.

Integrating Mindfulness into Daily Activities

Integrating mindfulness into daily activities is a powerful way to cultivate present-moment awareness, reduce stress, and promote holistic health and well-being. Here are some practical ways to incorporate mindfulness into your daily routine:

1. **Mindful Morning Routine:** Start your day with a mindful morning routine to set a positive tone for the day ahead. Begin by taking a few moments upon waking to focus on your breath and set an intention for the day. Engage in activities such as mindful stretching, meditation, or gratitude journaling to center yourself and cultivate a sense of presence and purpose.

2. **Mindful Eating:** Practice mindful eating by bringing awareness to the sensory experience of eating and savoring each bite of food. Turn off distractions such as screens and electronics, and take the time to fully engage your senses while eating. Notice the colors, textures, aromas,

and flavors of your food, and pay attention to hunger and fullness cues. Chew slowly and mindfully, and cultivate gratitude for the nourishment your food provides.

3. **Mindful Movement:** Incorporate mindful movement into your daily routine by engaging in activities such as yoga, tai chi, or walking meditation. Focus on the sensations of movement, breath, and energy flow as you move your body mindfully. Tune into the rhythm of your breath and the sensations in your muscles and joints, and allow yourself to be fully present in the moment.

4. **Mindful Work Habits:** Bring mindfulness to your workday by incorporating short mindfulness breaks throughout the day. Take a few moments to pause and breathe mindfully between tasks, and practice bringing your attention back to the present moment whenever you notice your mind wandering. Cultivate awareness of your thoughts, emotions, and bodily sensations as you engage in work-related activities, and practice responding with mindfulness rather than reacting impulsively.

5. **Mindful Communication:** Practice mindful communication by listening attentively to others with an open heart and mind. Pay attention to both verbal and non-verbal cues, and communicate with empathy, compassion, and authenticity. Be present with the person you are speaking to, and cultivate deep listening and understanding. Notice any automatic judgments or reactions that arise, and practice responding with mindfulness and intentionality.

6. **Mindful Evening Wind-Down:** Wind down your evening with a mindful bedtime routine to promote relaxation and prepare for restful sleep. Engage in activities such as gentle stretching, meditation, or reading, and create a calming environment free from screens and electronic devices. Reflect on the events of the day with compassion and acceptance, and practice gratitude for the moments of joy and connection you experienced.

7. **Mindful Daily Reflection:** Take time each day to reflect mindfully on your experiences, thoughts, and emotions. Journaling can be a helpful tool for processing and integrating your experiences, as well as

cultivating self-awareness and insight. Notice any patterns or recurring themes in your thoughts and emotions, and practice responding with mindfulness and self-compassion.

Chapter 4
Holistic Exercise and Movement

The Importance of Holistic Physical Activity

Holistic exercise and movement play a vital role in promoting overall well-being by addressing the interconnectedness of the mind, body, and spirit. Here's a look at the importance of holistic physical activity:

1. **Comprehensive Fitness:** Holistic exercise and movement encompass a variety of physical activities that engage the body in different ways, including cardiovascular exercise, strength training, flexibility exercises, balance and coordination drills, and mind-body practices such as yoga, tai chi, and qigong. By incorporating diverse movement modalities into your fitness routine, you can develop a well-rounded and comprehensive approach to physical fitness that supports overall health and vitality.

2. **Mind-Body Connection:** Holistic exercise and movement emphasize the integration of the mind and body, fostering greater awareness, presence, and mindfulness during physical activity. Mind-body practices such as yoga, tai chi, and mindful movement encourage conscious movement, breath awareness, and mental focus, promoting relaxation, stress reduction, and emotional well-being. By connecting the mind and body through movement, you can enhance your overall sense of balance, harmony, and inner peace.

3. **Functional Movement:** Holistic physical activity focuses on functional movement patterns that mimic real-life activities and promote optimal movement efficiency, mobility, and stability. Functional exercises such as squats, lunges, pushes, pulls, twists, and bends help improve posture, alignment, and joint integrity, reducing the risk of injury and enhancing everyday activities such as walking, bending, lifting, and reaching. By incorporating functional movement into your exercise routine, you can enhance your overall movement quality and resilience.

4. **Holistic Wellness:** Holistic exercise and movement support holistic wellness by addressing physical, mental, emotional, and spiritual aspects of health. Physical activity has been shown to improve cardiovascular health, muscular strength and endurance, bone density, flexibility, and metabolic function. Additionally, regular exercise can

enhance mood, reduce symptoms of anxiety and depression, boost cognitive function, and promote overall quality of life. By embracing holistic physical activity, you can nurture your body, mind, and spirit and cultivate a foundation for optimal well-being.

5. **Individualized Approach:** Holistic exercise and movement recognize that each person is unique and may have different needs, preferences, and abilities when it comes to physical activity. Rather than adhering to a one-size-fits-all approach, holistic fitness embraces individualized programming that takes into account factors such as age, fitness level, health status, goals, and interests. By tailoring your exercise routine to meet your specific needs and preferences, you can create a sustainable and enjoyable approach to physical activity that supports long-term adherence and success.

6. **Lifelong Health and Longevity:** Holistic exercise and movement promote lifelong health and longevity by supporting physical function, independence, and vitality as you age. Regular physical activity has been associated with numerous health benefits, including reduced risk of chronic diseases such as heart disease, diabetes, cancer, and osteoporosis, as well as improved longevity and quality of life. By making holistic physical activity a priority throughout your life, you can enhance your overall healthspan and enjoy a higher quality of life well into old age.

Mindful Movement Practices (Yoga, Tai Chi, Qigong)

Mindful movement practices such as yoga, Tai Chi, and Qigong are integral components of holistic exercise and movement, offering a unique blend of physical activity, breath awareness, and mindfulness. These practices promote balance, flexibility, strength, relaxation, and inner peace, fostering holistic health and well-being. Here's a closer look at each practice:

1. **Yoga:**
   - **Physical Benefits:** Yoga consists of a series of postures (asanas) that promote flexibility, strength, and balance. Practicing yoga can improve

muscular endurance, enhance joint mobility, and promote proper alignment and posture.

   - **Mental Benefits:** Yoga incorporates breath awareness and mindfulness techniques that help calm the mind, reduce stress, and promote relaxation. Regular yoga practice has been shown to improve mood, reduce symptoms of anxiety and depression, and enhance overall mental well-being.

   - **Spiritual Connection:** Yoga originated as a spiritual practice in ancient India and includes philosophical teachings that emphasize self-awareness, compassion, and unity. Many yoga traditions incorporate meditation, chanting, and other spiritual practices to deepen the practitioner's connection to their inner self and the larger universe.

2. Tai Chi:

   - **Physical Benefits:** Tai Chi is a gentle form of martial art characterized by slow, flowing movements and deep breathing. Practicing Tai Chi can improve balance, coordination, and flexibility while promoting relaxation and reducing tension in the body.

   - **Mental Benefits:** Tai Chi emphasizes mindfulness, concentration, and focused attention on the present moment. Practicing Tai Chi has been shown to improve cognitive function, enhance mental clarity, and reduce symptoms of stress and anxiety.

   - **Energy Flow:** Tai Chi incorporates the concept of Qi (pronounced "chee"), or life energy, and aims to promote the smooth flow of Qi throughout the body. By practicing Tai Chi, individuals can cultivate a sense of harmony and balance in both body and mind.

3. Qigong:

   - **Physical Benefits:** Qigong involves gentle movements, breathwork, and meditation to promote physical health and vitality. Practicing Qigong can improve balance, flexibility, and circulation while reducing tension and promoting relaxation in the body.

   - **Energetic Healing:** Qigong is rooted in Chinese medicine and the concept of Qi, or vital energy, which flows through the body along specific pathways called meridians. By practicing Qigong, individuals can cultivate and balance their Qi, promoting health and well-being on a physical, emotional, and energetic level.

   - **Mind-Body Connection:** Qigong emphasizes the connection between the mind, body, and spirit and aims to harmonize these aspects of the self. By practicing Qigong, individuals can develop greater self-awareness, inner peace, and a deeper sense of connection to themselves and the world around them.

Finding Joy in Exercise

Finding joy in exercise is essential for cultivating a sustainable and fulfilling approach to physical activity that supports holistic health and well-being. Here are some strategies for discovering joy in exercise:

1. **Choose Activities You Enjoy:** Select physical activities that you genuinely enjoy and look forward to. Whether it's hiking in nature, dancing to your favorite music, practicing yoga, playing a sport, or taking a group fitness class, find activities that bring you pleasure and fulfillment. Experiment with different types of exercise until you discover what resonates with you and makes you feel alive and energized.

2. **Focus on Fun and Playfulness:** Approach exercise with a sense of fun, playfulness, and curiosity. Embrace your inner child and engage in activities that make you feel joyful and lighthearted. Play games, try new sports or recreational activities, and challenge yourself to step outside your comfort zone. Remember that exercise doesn't have to be rigid or structured—it can be a playful and enjoyable way to move your body and express yourself.

3. **Connect with Nature:** Take advantage of outdoor environments and connect with nature as you exercise. Whether it's hiking in the mountains, swimming in the ocean, cycling through scenic trails, or practicing yoga in the park, spending time in nature can enhance your sense of well-being and bring a deeper sense of joy and appreciation to your workouts. Notice the sights, sounds, and sensations of the natural world as you move your body, and allow yourself to be fully present in the moment.

4. **Cultivate Mindfulness and Presence:** Practice mindfulness and presence as you exercise, bringing focused attention to the sensations of movement, breath, and energy flow in your body. Tune into the rhythm of your breath, the feeling of your muscles contracting and

releasing, and the sense of vitality and aliveness that arises when you move your body mindfully. By cultivating present-moment awareness, you can enhance the joy and satisfaction you experience during exercise.

5. **Set Realistic Goals and Expectations:** Set realistic goals and expectations for your exercise routine, focusing on progress rather than perfection. Celebrate your achievements, no matter how small, and acknowledge the effort and dedication you put into your workouts. Avoid comparing yourself to others or striving for unrealistic standards of fitness. Instead, focus on your own journey and embrace the process of growth and self-discovery.

6. **Find Social Support and Community:** Exercise with friends, family members, or like-minded individuals who share your interests and enthusiasm for physical activity. Join group fitness classes, sports teams, or outdoor recreation clubs to connect with others and foster a sense of camaraderie and support. Surround yourself with positive influences who inspire and motivate you to stay active and engaged in your fitness journey.

7. **Listen to Your Body:** Pay attention to your body's cues and honor your physical and emotional needs during exercise. Rest when you're tired, modify exercises as needed, and avoid pushing yourself beyond your limits. Exercise should feel invigorating and empowering, not draining or punishing. By listening to your body and honoring its signals, you can cultivate a more compassionate and sustainable approach to fitness.

8. **Celebrate Non-Scale Victories:** Shift your focus away from the scale and traditional measures of success, and instead celebrate non-scale victories and improvements in your overall well-being. Notice how exercise makes you feel stronger, more energetic, and more confident in your body. Celebrate improvements in your mood, stress levels, sleep quality, and overall quality of life as you prioritize regular physical activity.

Balancing Cardiovascular and Strength Training

Balancing cardiovascular and strength training is crucial for achieving a well-rounded and holistic approach to exercise that promotes overall health and well-being. Here are some key principles for integrating both types of training into your fitness routine:

1. Understanding Cardiovascular Exercise:

- **Definition:** Cardiovascular exercise, also known as aerobic exercise, involves activities that elevate your heart rate and increase your breathing rate over an extended period. Examples include running, cycling, swimming, brisk walking, and dancing.
- **Benefits:** Cardiovascular exercise improves cardiovascular health by strengthening the heart and lungs, enhancing circulation, and increasing endurance. It also helps burn calories, improve metabolism, and reduce the risk of chronic diseases such as heart disease, diabetes, and obesity.

2. Understanding Strength Training:

- **Definition:** Strength training, also known as resistance training or weight training, involves exercises that use resistance to build muscle strength, endurance, and power. This can be done using free weights, resistance bands, weight machines, or bodyweight exercises.
- **Benefits:** Strength training increases muscle mass, improves bone density, enhances joint stability, and boosts metabolism. It also helps improve functional strength, posture, and balance, reducing the risk of injury and enhancing overall physical performance.

3. Balancing Cardiovascular and Strength Training:

- **Frequency:** Aim to incorporate both cardiovascular and strength training into your weekly routine. A balanced approach may include 3-5 days of cardiovascular exercise and 2-3 days of strength training per week.
- **Variety:** Mix up your workouts to include a variety of cardiovascular and strength training activities. This can prevent boredom, challenge your body in different ways, and reduce the risk of overuse injuries.
- **Intensity:** Alternate between high-intensity and moderate-intensity workouts to challenge your cardiovascular system and build strength and endurance. Incorporate interval training, circuit training, and progressive overload techniques to continually challenge your body and see improvements in fitness.

- **Recovery:** Allow adequate time for rest and recovery between workouts, especially after intense strength training sessions. This allows your muscles to repair and rebuild stronger, reducing the risk of overtraining and injury.
- **Flexibility:** Don't forget to include flexibility exercises such as stretching, yoga, or Pilates in your routine to improve joint mobility, prevent muscle imbalances, and enhance overall flexibility and range of motion.

4. **Sample Workout Schedule:**
   - Monday: Cardiovascular exercise (e.g., running, cycling)
   - Tuesday: Strength training (e.g., full-body workout)
   - Wednesday: Rest or low-intensity activity (e.g., yoga, walking)
   - Thursday: Cardiovascular exercise (e.g., swimming, HIIT)
   - Friday: Strength training (e.g., upper body focus)
   - Saturday: Cardiovascular exercise (e.g., hiking, dance class)
   - Sunday: Rest or active recovery (e.g., stretching, leisurely bike ride)

5. **Listen to Your Body:**
   - Pay attention to how your body feels during and after exercise. If you experience pain, discomfort, or excessive fatigue, adjust your workout intensity or duration accordingly.
   - Stay hydrated, fuel your body with nutritious foods, and prioritize sleep and recovery to support your fitness goals and overall well-being.

Customizing Exercise for Individual Needs

Customizing exercise for individual needs is essential for promoting holistic health and well-being, as it allows individuals to tailor their fitness routines to their unique goals, preferences, abilities, and limitations. Here are some strategies for customizing exercise to meet individual needs:

1. **Assessing Personal Goals and Objectives:**
   - Begin by identifying your personal health and fitness goals. Whether you aim to improve cardiovascular health, build strength and muscle tone, increase flexibility, manage weight, reduce stress, or enhance

overall well-being, clarifying your objectives will help guide your exercise choices and program design.

2. Understanding Individual Preferences and Interests:
   - Consider your preferences and interests when selecting exercise activities. If you enjoy outdoor activities, consider hiking, cycling, or gardening. If you prefer group settings, explore options such as group fitness classes or team sports. Choose activities that you genuinely enjoy and look forward to, as this will increase motivation and adherence to your fitness routine.

3. Accounting for Physical Abilities and Limitations:
   - Take into account your current fitness level, physical abilities, and any limitations or medical conditions you may have. If you have existing injuries or health concerns, consult with a healthcare professional or qualified fitness trainer to develop a safe and effective exercise plan that accommodates your needs and minimizes the risk of injury.

4. Tailoring Exercise Intensity and Duration:
   - Customize the intensity and duration of your workouts based on your fitness level and goals. If you're new to exercise or returning after a period of inactivity, start gradually and progress slowly to avoid overexertion and injury. Listen to your body and adjust the intensity, duration, and frequency of your workouts as needed to ensure they remain challenging yet manageable.

5. Choosing Appropriate Exercise Modalities:
   - Select exercise modalities that align with your goals, preferences, and physical abilities. Whether you prefer cardiovascular activities such as walking, jogging, swimming, or cycling, or strength training exercises using free weights, resistance bands, or bodyweight, choose modalities that suit your individual needs and preferences.

6. Incorporating Variety and Progression:
   - Keep your exercise routine varied and engaging by incorporating a mix of different activities and modalities. This not only prevents boredom but also challenges your body in different ways, leading to more comprehensive fitness gains. Additionally, progressively increase

the intensity, duration, or complexity of your workouts over time to continue seeing improvements in strength, endurance, and overall fitness.

7. Listening to Your Body:

- Pay attention to how your body responds to exercise and adjust your routine accordingly. If you experience pain, discomfort, or excessive fatigue, modify your workouts or seek guidance from a qualified fitness professional. Remember to prioritize rest, recovery, and self-care to prevent overtraining and promote optimal recovery between workouts.

8. Monitoring Progress and Adjusting Accordingly:

- Regularly assess your progress towards your fitness goals and make adjustments to your exercise routine as needed. Keep track of key metrics such as strength gains, endurance improvements, changes in body composition, and overall well-being. Celebrate your achievements and be flexible in adapting your routine to accommodate changes in your goals, preferences, and lifestyle.

Chapter 5
Holistic Approaches to Mental Health

Holistic Strategies for Mental Well-Being

Holistic approaches to mental well-being encompass a range of strategies that address the interconnectedness of the mind, body, and spirit to promote overall mental health and emotional balance. Here are some holistic strategies for enhancing mental well-being:

1. Mindfulness and Meditation:
   - Practice mindfulness meditation to cultivate present-moment awareness, reduce stress, and enhance emotional resilience. Set aside time each day to engage in mindfulness practices such as breath awareness, body scanning, or loving-kindness meditation. Regular meditation can help calm the mind, improve focus, and foster a sense of inner peace and well-being.

2. Physical Activity and Exercise:
   - Engage in regular physical activity and exercise to boost mood, reduce symptoms of anxiety and depression, and improve overall mental health. Choose activities that you enjoy, whether it's walking, jogging, cycling, yoga, or dancing, and aim for at least 30 minutes of moderate-intensity exercise most days of the week. Physical activity releases endorphins, neurotransmitters that promote feelings of happiness and well-being, and can serve as a powerful antidote to stress and negative emotions.

3. Nutrition and Diet:
   - Adopt a balanced and nourishing diet that supports optimal brain function and mental health. Focus on whole, nutrient-dense foods such as fruits, vegetables, whole grains, lean proteins, and healthy fats. Incorporate foods rich in omega-3 fatty acids, such as salmon, walnuts, and flaxseeds, which have been linked to improved mood and cognitive function. Limit consumption of processed foods, refined sugars, and alcohol, which can negatively impact mood and mental well-being.

4. Quality Sleep:
   - Prioritize quality sleep as a cornerstone of mental health and well-being. Aim for 7-9 hours of restful sleep each night and establish a regular sleep schedule to regulate your body's internal clock. Create a relaxing bedtime routine to signal to your body that it's time to wind

down, such as taking a warm bath, practicing relaxation techniques, or reading a book. Ensure your sleep environment is comfortable, quiet, and conducive to restorative sleep.

5. Stress Management:

   - Develop effective stress management techniques to cope with life's challenges and reduce the impact of stress on mental health. Practice relaxation techniques such as deep breathing, progressive muscle relaxation, or guided imagery to activate the body's relaxation response and counteract the effects of stress. Prioritize self-care activities that promote relaxation and rejuvenation, such as spending time in nature, practicing hobbies, or connecting with loved ones.

6. Social Connection:

   - Cultivate meaningful social connections and nurturing relationships to support mental well-being. Spend time with family and friends, engage in social activities and group gatherings, and seek out supportive communities or support groups. Strong social connections provide a sense of belonging, validation, and emotional support, buffering against feelings of loneliness, isolation, and depression.

7. Mind-Body Therapies:

   - Explore mind-body therapies such as yoga, tai chi, qigong, acupuncture, and massage therapy, which integrate physical, mental, and emotional elements to promote holistic healing. These therapies can help reduce stress, improve mood, enhance relaxation, and restore balance to the mind and body.

8. Creative Expression and Self-Discovery:

   - Engage in creative expression and self-discovery activities to foster self-awareness, self-expression, and personal growth. Explore artistic pursuits such as painting, writing, music, or dance, or try journaling, visualization, or expressive therapies to explore your thoughts, feelings, and innermost desires.

Emotional Resilience and Coping Mechanisms

Emotional resilience and coping mechanisms are essential components of holistic approaches to mental health, empowering individuals to navigate life's challenges, manage stress, and bounce back from adversity. Here are some strategies for building emotional resilience and cultivating effective coping mechanisms:

1. **Develop Self-Awareness:**
   - Cultivate self-awareness by paying attention to your thoughts, emotions, and reactions to different situations. Notice patterns in your behavior and identify triggers for stress, anxiety, or negative emotions. By becoming more aware of your internal experiences, you can gain insight into your emotional responses and develop strategies for managing them effectively.

2. **Practice Mindfulness:**
   - Engage in mindfulness practices to cultivate present-moment awareness and non-judgmental acceptance of your thoughts and feelings. Mindfulness meditation, deep breathing exercises, and body scan techniques can help anchor you in the present moment, reduce rumination, and promote emotional regulation. Regular mindfulness practice can enhance your ability to cope with stress and cultivate a greater sense of inner peace and resilience.

3. **Build Strong Social Support:**
   - Foster supportive relationships with friends, family members, and peers who provide emotional validation, empathy, and understanding. Reach out to trusted individuals for support during difficult times, and be willing to offer support to others in return. Strong social connections provide a buffer against stress, loneliness, and isolation, enhancing emotional resilience and well-being.

4. **Develop Healthy Coping Strategies:**
   - Identify healthy coping strategies that help you manage stress and regulate your emotions in constructive ways. This may include engaging in physical activity, practicing relaxation techniques, journaling, creative expression, or spending time in nature. Experiment with different coping strategies to find what works best for you and incorporate them into your daily routine.

5. **Cultivate Optimism and Positive Thinking:**
   - Foster a positive outlook on life by focusing on gratitude, hope, and optimism. Practice reframing negative thoughts and beliefs into more positive and empowering perspectives. Cultivate gratitude by keeping a gratitude journal and reflecting on the things you appreciate in your life. Developing a resilient mindset can help you navigate challenges with greater resilience and adaptability.

6. **Set Realistic Goals and Expectations:**
   - Establish realistic goals and expectations for yourself, taking into account your abilities, resources, and limitations. Break larger goals into smaller, manageable steps, and celebrate your progress along the way. By setting achievable goals and acknowledging your accomplishments, you can build confidence and resilience in the face of adversity.

7. **Seek Professional Support When Needed:**
   - Don't hesitate to seek professional support from therapists, counselors, or mental health professionals if you're struggling to cope with difficult emotions or life circumstances. Therapy can provide a safe and supportive space to explore your feelings, gain new perspectives, and develop effective coping strategies. Asking for help is a sign of strength and courage, and reaching out for support can empower you to overcome challenges and thrive.

8. **Practice Self-Care and Stress Management:**
   - Prioritize self-care practices that nurture your physical, mental, and emotional well-being. This may include getting adequate sleep, eating a balanced diet, engaging in regular physical activity, and practicing relaxation techniques such as yoga, meditation, or deep breathing exercises. Set boundaries to protect your time and energy, and prioritize activities that replenish and rejuvenate you.

Mind-Body Therapies for Mental Health

Mind-body therapies offer holistic approaches to mental health by integrating the interconnectedness of the mind, body, and spirit to promote overall well-being. These therapies recognize the profound influence of mental and emotional states on physical health and vice versa, and they utilize various techniques to support mental health and emotional balance. Here are several mind-body therapies commonly used for mental health:

1. Yoga:
- **Description:** Yoga is a mind-body practice that combines physical postures, breathwork, meditation, and relaxation techniques to promote holistic health and well-being. There are many styles of yoga, ranging from gentle and restorative to vigorous and dynamic.
- **Benefits:** Yoga has been shown to reduce stress, anxiety, and depression by calming the nervous system, promoting relaxation, and increasing self-awareness. Regular practice of yoga can improve mood, enhance emotional resilience, and foster a sense of inner peace and well-being.

2. Tai Chi:
- **Description:** Tai Chi is a gentle form of martial art characterized by slow, flowing movements and deep breathing. It emphasizes mindfulness, balance, and the integration of mind and body.
- **Benefits:** Tai Chi has been shown to reduce stress, anxiety, and depression by promoting relaxation, improving mood, and enhancing mental clarity. The slow, deliberate movements of Tai Chi can help calm the mind, reduce muscle tension, and increase energy flow throughout the body.

3. Qigong:
- **Description:** Qigong is a holistic mind-body practice that integrates physical movement, breathwork, meditation, and visualization to promote health and vitality. It is rooted in Chinese medicine and philosophy and is based on the concept of Qi, or vital energy.
- **Benefits:** Qigong has been shown to reduce stress, anxiety, and depression by promoting relaxation, balancing energy flow, and harmonizing the mind and body. Regular practice of Qigong can improve mood, increase resilience to stress, and enhance overall well-being.

4. Mindfulness-Based Stress Reduction (MBSR):

- **Description:** MBSR is a structured program that incorporates mindfulness meditation, gentle yoga, and awareness practices to reduce stress, enhance self-awareness, and promote well-being. It was developed by Dr. Jon Kabat-Zinn at the University of Massachusetts Medical School.

- **Benefits:** MBSR has been extensively researched and shown to be effective in reducing symptoms of stress, anxiety, depression, and chronic pain. By cultivating present-moment awareness and non-judgmental acceptance, MBSR helps individuals develop greater resilience and coping skills in the face of life's challenges.

5. Biofeedback:

- **Description:** Biofeedback is a mind-body therapy that uses electronic monitoring devices to provide real-time feedback on physiological processes such as heart rate, muscle tension, and skin temperature. By learning to control these physiological responses, individuals can reduce stress and improve mental and emotional well-being.

- **Benefits:** Biofeedback has been used to treat a variety of mental health conditions, including anxiety disorders, depression, and PTSD. By increasing awareness of physiological responses and learning relaxation techniques, individuals can gain greater control over their stress responses and improve their overall mental health.

6. Breathwork:

- **Description:** Breathwork encompasses various techniques for conscious breathing, such as diaphragmatic breathing, deep breathing, and rhythmic breathing. These techniques can help regulate the autonomic nervous system, reduce stress, and promote relaxation.

- **Benefits:** Breathwork has been shown to reduce symptoms of anxiety, depression, and PTSD by activating the body's relaxation response and calming the mind. By focusing on the breath, individuals can increase self-awareness, reduce rumination, and cultivate a greater sense of inner peace and well-being.

7. Guided Imagery and Visualization:

- **Description:** Guided imagery and visualization involve using mental imagery and imagination to evoke positive sensations, emotions, and experiences. This can be done individually or with the guidance of a therapist or audio recording.

- **Benefits:** Guided imagery and visualization have been shown to reduce stress, anxiety, and depression by promoting relaxation, improving mood, and enhancing self-regulation skills. By creating vivid mental images of healing and well-being, individuals can tap into their innate capacity for self-healing and transformation.

Nurturing Healthy Relationships for Emotional Wellness

Nurturing healthy relationships is a fundamental aspect of holistic approaches to mental health, as supportive connections with others play a crucial role in promoting emotional wellness and overall well-being. Here are several strategies for cultivating and sustaining healthy relationships for emotional wellness:

1. **Effective Communication:**
   - Foster open, honest, and respectful communication with your loved ones. Practice active listening, empathy, and validation to understand and acknowledge each other's thoughts, feelings, and perspectives. Communicate your own needs, boundaries, and concerns openly and assertively, and encourage others to do the same.

2. **Establishing Boundaries:**
   - Set clear boundaries in your relationships to protect your emotional well-being and ensure mutual respect and understanding. Identify your personal limits, preferences, and values, and communicate them assertively to others. Respect the boundaries of others and honor their needs and preferences as well.

3. **Building Trust and Mutual Support:**
   - Cultivate trust, reliability, and dependability in your relationships by following through on commitments, being consistent in your actions, and demonstrating honesty and integrity. Offer emotional support, encouragement, and validation to your loved ones during times of difficulty, and be willing to seek support from others when needed.

4. **Conflict Resolution Skills:**

- Develop effective conflict resolution skills to navigate disagreements and conflicts in a constructive and respectful manner. Practice active listening, empathy, and problem-solving techniques to address differences and find mutually satisfactory solutions. Approach conflicts with an attitude of curiosity, openness, and willingness to compromise.

5. Quality Time Together:
- Prioritize quality time spent together with your loved ones to strengthen your bonds and foster emotional connection. Engage in shared activities, hobbies, or interests that bring you joy and fulfillment, and create opportunities for meaningful conversations and shared experiences. Show appreciation and affection for each other through gestures of kindness, affection, and gratitude.

6. Cultivating Empathy and Compassion:
- Cultivate empathy, compassion, and understanding in your relationships by acknowledging and validating each other's emotions and experiences. Practice empathy by putting yourself in the shoes of others and seeking to understand their perspectives and feelings. Offer support, encouragement, and kindness to your loved ones, even in times of disagreement or conflict.

7. Healthy Conflict Resolution:
- Learn to manage conflicts and disagreements in a healthy and constructive manner. Avoid criticism, defensiveness, and blame, and instead focus on expressing your feelings and needs assertively and listening actively to the perspective of the other person. Use "I" statements to communicate your thoughts and feelings without assigning blame, and work together to find mutually acceptable solutions.

8. Seeking Support When Needed:
- Recognize when you need support and seek help from trusted friends, family members, or mental health professionals. Reach out for support during challenging times, transitions, or crises, and be willing to offer support to others in return. Building a network of supportive relationships can provide a source of strength, resilience, and comfort during difficult times.

The Role of Spirituality in Mental Well-Being

The role of spirituality in mental well-being is significant, as it provides individuals with a sense of meaning, purpose, and connection to something greater than themselves. Spirituality encompasses beliefs, values, practices, and experiences related to the search for transcendent meaning and inner peace. Here are several ways in which spirituality can contribute to mental well-being:

1. **Finding Meaning and Purpose:**
   - Spirituality offers a framework for exploring existential questions and finding meaning and purpose in life. Beliefs in a higher power, divine purpose, or interconnectedness with the universe can provide individuals with a sense of direction, fulfillment, and significance, even in the face of adversity or uncertainty.

2. **Enhancing Resilience and Coping Skills:**
   - Spirituality can enhance resilience and coping skills by providing individuals with a source of strength, hope, and inner peace during difficult times. Spiritual practices such as prayer, meditation, and mindfulness can help individuals develop greater emotional resilience, acceptance, and equanimity in the face of life's challenges.

3. **Promoting Emotional Regulation:**
   - Spiritual practices and beliefs can promote emotional regulation by providing individuals with tools and resources for managing stress, anxiety, and other negative emotions. Practices such as meditation, yoga, and breathwork can help calm the mind, reduce physiological arousal, and promote relaxation and emotional balance.

4. **Fostering Connection and Community:**
   - Spirituality fosters connection and community by providing individuals with opportunities to connect with like-minded individuals, share common beliefs and values, and engage in supportive relationships. Spiritual communities such as churches, temples, mosques, or meditation groups can offer a sense of belonging,

acceptance, and social support, which are essential for mental well-being.

5. Cultivating Compassion and Empathy:
- Spirituality encourages the cultivation of compassion, empathy, and altruism towards oneself and others. Beliefs in interconnectedness, universal love, and the inherent worth and dignity of all beings can inspire individuals to act with kindness, generosity, and compassion, fostering greater emotional well-being and social connection.

6. Providing a Source of Comfort and Hope:
- Spirituality can provide individuals with a source of comfort, solace, and hope during times of grief, loss, or despair. Beliefs in an afterlife, divine grace, or the ultimate goodness of the universe can offer reassurance and perspective, helping individuals find meaning and purpose in their suffering and resilience in the face of adversity.

7. Facilitating Self-Discovery and Growth:
- Spirituality facilitates self-discovery and personal growth by encouraging individuals to explore their innermost beliefs, values, and aspirations. Practices such as meditation, journaling, and contemplative reflection can help individuals deepen their self-awareness, cultivate self-compassion, and align their actions with their core values and aspirations.

8. Promoting Forgiveness and Healing:
- Spirituality promotes forgiveness, reconciliation, and healing by encouraging individuals to let go of resentment, bitterness, and grudges towards themselves and others. Beliefs in divine forgiveness, grace, and redemption can offer individuals a sense of liberation, peace, and wholeness, facilitating emotional healing and reconciliation in relationships.

Chapter 6
Holistic Healing Modalities

Acupuncture and Traditional Chinese Medicine

Acupuncture and Traditional Chinese Medicine (TCM) are holistic healing modalities that have been practiced for thousands of years, originating in ancient China. These modalities are based on the concept of balancing the flow of vital energy, or Qi (pronounced "chee"), within the body to promote health and well-being. Here's an overview of acupuncture and TCM:

1. **Acupuncture:**
   - **Description:** Acupuncture is a therapeutic technique that involves inserting thin needles into specific points on the body to stimulate and balance the flow of Qi along energy pathways known as meridians. The goal of acupuncture is to restore harmony and balance within the body, mind, and spirit.
   - **Principles:** According to TCM principles, illness and disease result from imbalances or blockages in the flow of Qi through the meridians. By inserting acupuncture needles into specific points along the meridians, practitioners aim to restore the smooth flow of Qi, promote circulation, and stimulate the body's natural healing mechanisms.
   - **Conditions Treated:** Acupuncture is used to treat a wide range of physical, emotional, and psychological conditions, including pain, inflammation, digestive disorders, respiratory conditions, hormonal imbalances, stress, anxiety, depression, and insomnia. It is often used as part of an integrative approach to healthcare, complementing conventional medical treatments.

2. **Traditional Chinese Medicine (TCM):**
   - **Description:** TCM is a comprehensive system of healing that encompasses various modalities, including acupuncture, herbal medicine, dietary therapy, massage (Tui Na), cupping, and qigong. TCM views health as a state of balance and harmony between the body's internal organs, systems, and energies.
   - **Principles:** TCM is based on the principles of Yin and Yang, the Five Elements (Wood, Fire, Earth, Metal, Water), and the concept of Qi and Blood. Health is seen as a dynamic equilibrium between these opposing forces, and illness arises when there is an imbalance or disharmony between them. TCM treatments aim to restore balance and harmony by

addressing the root cause of illness and supporting the body's innate healing capacity.

- **Approach to Diagnosis:** TCM practitioners use a holistic approach to diagnosis, taking into account a person's constitution, lifestyle, emotional state, and environmental factors in addition to their symptoms. Diagnostic techniques may include observation, palpation, questioning, and pulse and tongue diagnosis.

- **Conditions Treated:** TCM can effectively treat a wide range of acute and chronic health conditions, including digestive disorders, respiratory conditions, musculoskeletal pain, gynecological issues, skin disorders, and emotional imbalances. TCM treatments are tailored to the individual's unique pattern of disharmony and may involve a combination of acupuncture, herbal medicine, dietary and lifestyle recommendations, and other therapeutic modalities.

3. **Integration with Conventional Medicine:**

- Acupuncture and TCM are increasingly being integrated into conventional healthcare settings as complementary therapies to support overall health and wellness. Many healthcare providers recognize the value of these holistic modalities in addressing a variety of health concerns and promoting holistic healing.

- Research continues to explore the mechanisms of acupuncture and TCM and their efficacy in treating various conditions. Numerous studies have shown positive outcomes for acupuncture in pain management, stress reduction, and other health issues, contributing to its growing acceptance and popularity in mainstream medicine.

Ayurveda: The Science of Life

Ayurveda, often referred to as "The Science of Life," is a holistic healing system that originated in ancient India over 5,000 years ago. It offers a comprehensive approach to health and wellness, focusing on the interconnectedness of the body, mind, and spirit. Here's an overview of Ayurveda and its key principles:

1. **Principles of Ayurveda:**
- **Doshas:** Ayurveda is based on the principle of the three doshas—Vata, Pitta, and Kapha—which are biological energies that govern

various physiological and psychological functions in the body. Each individual has a unique constitution, or prakriti, which is determined by the dominant doshas.

- **Balance:** Health in Ayurveda is defined as a state of balance and harmony between the doshas, with each person striving to maintain their unique constitutional balance. Imbalances or disturbances in the doshas can lead to disease and dysfunction.

- **Dhatus and Malas:** Ayurveda also recognizes the importance of the dhatus (tissues) and malas (waste products) in maintaining health. Proper digestion, absorption, and elimination are essential for the production of healthy tissues and the removal of toxins from the body.

2. Diagnostic Techniques:

- **Pulse Diagnosis:** Ayurvedic practitioners use pulse diagnosis, or Nadi Pariksha, to assess the balance of the doshas and identify imbalances or disturbances in the body. By feeling the pulse at various points on the wrist, practitioners can gather information about the state of the organs and systems.

- **Tongue Diagnosis:** Examination of the tongue's color, coating, shape, and texture can provide insights into the individual's digestive health, doshic balance, and overall well-being.

- **Observation and Inquiry:** Ayurvedic practitioners also rely on observation and inquiry to gather information about the individual's lifestyle, dietary habits, emotional state, and environmental influences. This comprehensive approach allows for a thorough assessment of the person's health status and potential imbalances.

3. Treatment Modalities:

- **Diet and Nutrition:** Ayurveda emphasizes the importance of diet and nutrition in maintaining health and preventing disease. Dietary recommendations are tailored to the individual's constitution, imbalances, and specific health concerns. Foods are classified according to their tastes, qualities, and effects on the doshas, and dietary guidelines focus on promoting balance and harmony within the body.

- **Herbal Medicine:** Ayurvedic herbs and herbal formulations are used to support the body's natural healing processes, restore balance to the doshas, and address specific health issues. Herbs are selected based on their taste, potency, and therapeutic properties, and may be used internally or externally in the form of powders, teas, oils, or pastes.

- **Yoga and Meditation:** Yoga and meditation are integral components of Ayurveda, promoting physical, mental, and spiritual well-being. Yoga practices such as asanas (postures), pranayama (breath control), and meditation help balance the doshas, improve digestion, enhance circulation, and reduce stress, anxiety, and mental agitation.
- **Panchakarma:** Panchakarma is a cleansing and detoxification therapy that involves a series of specialized treatments designed to remove toxins, impurities, and excess doshas from the body. These treatments may include oil massage (abhyanga), herbal steam therapy (swedana), nasal cleansing (nasya), therapeutic vomiting (vamana), purgation (virechana), and enemas (basti).
- **Lifestyle Recommendations:** Ayurveda offers lifestyle recommendations tailored to the individual's doshic constitution and specific health needs. These recommendations may include daily routines (dinacharya), seasonal routines (ritucharya), and guidelines for sleep, exercise, stress management, and self-care practices.

4. Holistic Approach to Health and Wellness:
- Ayurveda takes a holistic approach to health and wellness, addressing the physical, mental, emotional, and spiritual aspects of the individual. It recognizes the interconnectedness of all aspects of life and promotes balance and harmony within the body, mind, and spirit.
- By supporting the body's innate healing intelligence and addressing the root causes of disease, Ayurveda empowers individuals to take an active role in their health and well-being. It emphasizes preventive healthcare measures, lifestyle modifications, and self-care practices to maintain optimal health and vitality throughout life.

Naturopathy and Herbal Medicine

Naturopathy and herbal medicine are holistic healing modalities that emphasize the body's innate ability to heal itself and promote overall health and wellness through natural and non-invasive interventions. Here's an overview of naturopathy and herbal medicine:

1. Naturopathy:
- **Description:** Naturopathy is a holistic approach to healthcare that focuses on identifying and addressing the root causes of illness, rather

than just treating symptoms. Naturopathic doctors (NDs) use a combination of natural therapies, lifestyle interventions, and traditional healing modalities to support the body's inherent healing capacity.

- **Principles:** Naturopathy is guided by six fundamental principles, including the healing power of nature, identifying and treating the root cause, treating the whole person, supporting the body's self-healing mechanisms, emphasizing prevention, and doctor as teacher. These principles form the foundation of naturopathic philosophy and guide the practice of naturopathic medicine.

- **Treatment Modalities:** Naturopathic treatments may include dietary and nutritional counseling, herbal medicine, homeopathy, hydrotherapy, physical medicine, acupuncture, lifestyle counseling, and stress management techniques. Treatment plans are individualized based on the patient's unique needs, preferences, and health goals.

- **Conditions Treated:** Naturopathic medicine can effectively address a wide range of acute and chronic health conditions, including digestive disorders, hormonal imbalances, allergies, autoimmune diseases, musculoskeletal pain, cardiovascular conditions, mental health concerns, and chronic stress. Naturopathic doctors focus on restoring balance and optimizing health in all areas of the body, mind, and spirit.

2. Herbal Medicine:

- **Description:** Herbal medicine, also known as botanical medicine or phytotherapy, is the use of plants and plant-derived substances to prevent and treat illness and promote health and well-being. Herbal medicine has been used for thousands of years by cultures around the world and continues to be a central component of traditional healing systems.

- **Principles:** Herbal medicine is based on the principles of using whole plants or plant extracts to harness their therapeutic properties and synergistic effects. Herbs contain a wide array of bioactive compounds, including phytochemicals, antioxidants, vitamins, minerals, and essential oils, which have specific actions on the body's physiological functions.

- **Herbal Preparations:** Herbal remedies can be prepared in various forms, including teas, tinctures, capsules, tablets, extracts, poultices, salves, and essential oils. Each form of preparation has its unique advantages and may be chosen based on the herb's properties, intended use, and individual preferences.

- **Conditions Treated:** Herbal medicine can be used to treat a broad spectrum of health conditions, including digestive disorders, respiratory conditions, skin conditions, hormonal imbalances, immune system support, stress management, and mental health concerns. Herbs are chosen based on their specific therapeutic actions and indications for each condition, as well as the individual's constitution and health status.

3. Safety and Efficacy:

- Naturopathy and herbal medicine are generally considered safe when used appropriately under the guidance of qualified healthcare practitioners. However, it's important to consult with a licensed naturopathic doctor or herbalist before starting any herbal remedies or naturopathic treatments, especially if you have pre-existing health conditions, are taking medications, or are pregnant or breastfeeding.

- While herbal medicine offers many benefits, it's essential to use caution and follow recommended dosages and precautions to minimize the risk of adverse effects or interactions. Some herbs may interact with medications or exacerbate certain health conditions, so it's important to inform your healthcare provider of any herbal supplements you are taking.

4. Integration with Conventional Medicine:

- Naturopathy and herbal medicine are increasingly being integrated into conventional healthcare settings as complementary therapies to support overall health and wellness. Many healthcare providers recognize the value of these holistic modalities in addressing a variety of health concerns and promoting holistic healing.

- Research continues to explore the safety and efficacy of naturopathic treatments and herbal remedies for various health conditions. Numerous studies have shown promising results for the use of herbal medicine in managing pain, inflammation, digestive disorders, respiratory conditions, and mental health concerns, contributing to their growing acceptance and popularity in mainstream medicine.

Energy Healing Practices (Reiki, Healing Touch)

Energy healing practices such as Reiki and Healing Touch are holistic modalities that work with the body's subtle energy systems to promote physical, emotional, and spiritual well-being. These practices are based on the concept that the human body is surrounded by an energy field that can be influenced and manipulated to facilitate healing. Here's an overview of Reiki and Healing Touch:

1. **Reiki:**
   - **Description:** Reiki is a Japanese form of energy healing that was developed in the early 20th century by Mikao Usui. The word "Reiki" translates to "universal life energy," and the practice involves channeling this healing energy through the hands of the practitioner to the recipient. Reiki is based on the belief that when the body's energy is balanced and flowing freely, it can heal itself on physical, emotional, and spiritual levels.
   - **Principles:** Reiki is guided by five principles or precepts that promote harmony, peace, and spiritual growth. These principles include:
     1. Just for today, I will not be angry.
     2. Just for today, I will not worry.
     3. Just for today, I will be grateful.
     4. Just for today, I will do my work honestly.
     5. Just for today, I will be kind to every living thing.
   - **Techniques:** During a Reiki session, the practitioner places their hands lightly on or just above the recipient's body, focusing on specific energy centers known as chakras or areas of tension or discomfort. The practitioner acts as a channel for Reiki energy, allowing it to flow through their hands to the recipient. Reiki energy is believed to have an intelligent, healing effect on the body, promoting relaxation, stress reduction, pain relief, and overall well-being.
   - **Benefits:** Reiki is used to promote relaxation, reduce stress and anxiety, alleviate pain, support emotional healing, and enhance overall health and well-being. Many people report feeling a sense of deep relaxation, peace, and warmth during and after Reiki sessions, as well as improvements in physical symptoms and emotional balance.

2. **Healing Touch:**

- **Description**: Healing Touch is a holistic energy therapy that was developed in the late 20th century by Janet Mentgen, a nurse and holistic health educator. It is based on the premise that the human body has an energy field that can be influenced and manipulated to promote healing and well-being. Healing Touch incorporates techniques from various energy healing traditions, including Reiki, therapeutic touch, and qigong.
  - **Principles**: Healing Touch is guided by a set of principles that emphasize the importance of intention, compassion, and respect for the individual's innate healing capacity. Practitioners focus on creating a therapeutic relationship with the recipient and facilitating the body's natural healing process.
  - **Techniques**: Healing Touch techniques include gentle touch, manipulation of the energy field, visualization, and intention-setting. Practitioners work with the recipient's energy field to clear blockages, balance energy centers, and promote relaxation and healing. Healing Touch sessions may be tailored to address specific physical, emotional, or spiritual concerns.
  - **Benefits**: Healing Touch is used to support overall health and well-being, reduce stress and anxiety, alleviate pain, enhance immune function, accelerate wound healing, and promote emotional and spiritual growth. Many people report feeling a sense of deep relaxation, peace, and connection during and after Healing Touch sessions, as well as improvements in physical symptoms and emotional balance.

3. Integration with Conventional Medicine:

- Both Reiki and Healing Touch are increasingly being integrated into conventional healthcare settings as complementary therapies to support overall health and wellness. Many healthcare providers recognize the value of these holistic modalities in promoting relaxation, reducing stress, and enhancing the body's natural healing processes.
  - Research continues to explore the mechanisms of action and efficacy of Reiki and Healing Touch for various health conditions. While scientific evidence is still emerging, many studies have shown promising results for the use of energy healing practices in improving physical symptoms, emotional well-being, and quality of life, contributing to their growing acceptance and popularity in mainstream medicine.

Integrating Complementary Therapies for Holistic Healing

Integrating complementary therapies for holistic healing involves combining conventional medical treatments with alternative and complementary modalities to address the physical, emotional, and spiritual aspects of health and well-being. This approach recognizes that optimal health and wellness require a comprehensive and individualized approach that considers the whole person. Here's an overview of how complementary therapies can be integrated for holistic healing:

1. Collaborative Care:
   - Integrative healthcare involves collaboration between conventional medical providers, such as physicians, nurses, and specialists, and complementary healthcare practitioners, such as naturopathic doctors, acupuncturists, chiropractors, and massage therapists. By working together, healthcare providers can offer patients a broader range of treatment options and support their holistic healing journey.

2. Individualized Treatment Plans:
   - Integrative healthcare practitioners tailor treatment plans to each individual's unique needs, preferences, and health goals. This may involve combining conventional medical treatments with complementary therapies such as acupuncture, herbal medicine, massage therapy, mind-body techniques, and energy healing practices. Treatment plans are personalized to address the root causes of health issues and support the body's innate healing capacity.

3. Comprehensive Assessment:
   - Integrative healthcare providers conduct thorough assessments that take into account the physical, emotional, mental, and spiritual aspects of health. This may involve gathering information about the individual's medical history, lifestyle factors, stressors, emotional well-being, dietary habits, sleep patterns, and social support network. By understanding the whole person, healthcare providers can develop comprehensive treatment plans that address underlying imbalances and promote holistic healing.

4. Multimodal Approach:

- Holistic healing often involves a multimodal approach that combines different therapeutic modalities to address the complex interplay of factors contributing to health and wellness. For example, a treatment plan for chronic pain may include a combination of conventional pain medications, physical therapy, acupuncture, massage therapy, and stress reduction techniques such as mindfulness meditation or yoga. By addressing physical, emotional, and lifestyle factors, integrative therapies can help individuals achieve better outcomes and improve their overall quality of life.

5. Focus on Prevention:

- Integrative healthcare emphasizes preventive measures and lifestyle interventions to promote long-term health and well-being. This may include dietary and nutritional counseling, stress management techniques, exercise programs, and mind-body practices such as meditation, yoga, or tai chi. By empowering individuals to make positive lifestyle changes, integrative healthcare can help prevent chronic diseases and promote optimal health and wellness.

6. Patient-Centered Care:

- Integrative healthcare places a strong emphasis on patient-centered care, involving patients in the decision-making process and empowering them to take an active role in their health and healing journey. This may involve educating patients about their treatment options, discussing the potential benefits and risks of different therapies, and supporting them in making informed decisions that align with their values and preferences.

7. Research and Evidence-Based Practice:

- Integrative healthcare is grounded in research and evidence-based practice, with a growing body of scientific literature supporting the efficacy and safety of complementary therapies for various health conditions. Integrative healthcare providers stay up-to-date on the latest research findings and use evidence-based approaches to inform their clinical practice and treatment recommendations.

Chapter 7
Holistic Dentistry and Oral Health

Understanding Holistic Dentistry Principles

Holistic dentistry, also known as biological or integrative dentistry, is a patient-centered approach to dental care that considers the impact of oral health on the overall health and well-being of the individual. It integrates traditional dental practices with complementary and alternative therapies to promote holistic health and wellness. Here are the key principles of holistic dentistry:

1. **Whole-Person Approach:**
   - Holistic dentistry views the mouth as an integral part of the whole body and recognizes the interconnectedness of oral health with overall health and well-being. It considers how dental treatments and oral health practices may affect other systems of the body and vice versa.

2. **Biocompatibility of Dental Materials:**
   - Holistic dentistry emphasizes the use of biocompatible dental materials that are safe for the body and minimize potential adverse reactions. This includes avoiding the use of materials containing mercury, such as dental amalgam fillings, and opting for alternatives such as composite resin or porcelain restorations.

3. **Preventive and Minimally Invasive Approaches:**
   - Holistic dentistry focuses on preventive measures and minimally invasive treatments to preserve natural tooth structure and promote long-term oral health. This may include regular dental cleanings and exams, fluoride-free preventive treatments, sealants, and dietary counseling to minimize the risk of dental decay and gum disease.

4. **Mercury-Free Dentistry:**
   - Holistic dentistry advocates for the elimination of mercury-containing dental materials, such as dental amalgam fillings, due to concerns about potential health risks associated with mercury exposure. Instead, holistic dentists use mercury-free alternatives, such as composite resin or porcelain fillings, for dental restorations.

5. **Biological Compatibility Testing:**
   - Some holistic dentists offer biological compatibility testing to assess how the body may react to dental materials and treatments. These

tests may involve evaluating immune responses to dental materials or assessing genetic factors that may influence individual sensitivities.

6. Nutritional Counseling:

- Holistic dentistry recognizes the importance of nutrition in maintaining optimal oral health and overall well-being. Holistic dentists may provide nutritional counseling to support a healthy diet that promotes strong teeth and gums, minimizes the risk of dental decay and gum disease, and supports systemic health.

7. Integration of Complementary Therapies:

- Holistic dentistry integrates complementary and alternative therapies into dental care to support the body's natural healing processes and promote overall health and wellness. This may include techniques such as acupuncture, homeopathy, herbal medicine, ozone therapy, and energy healing practices.

8. Environmental Awareness:

- Holistic dentistry considers the environmental impact of dental practices and seeks to minimize the use of environmentally harmful materials and procedures. This may involve implementing eco-friendly practices, reducing waste and pollution, and using sustainable materials whenever possible.

9. Collaboration with Healthcare Providers:

- Holistic dentists collaborate with other healthcare providers, such as physicians, naturopathic doctors, and nutritionists, to provide comprehensive care that addresses the individual's overall health and wellness needs. This interdisciplinary approach ensures that all aspects of the patient's health are taken into consideration.

The Connection Between Oral Health and Overall Well-Being

The connection between oral health and overall well-being is profound, with research continually highlighting how the health of your mouth

can significantly impact your body's overall health. Here's an overview
of the relationship between oral health and overall well-being:

1. Systemic Health Impacts:

- Oral health is linked to various systemic health conditions, including
cardiovascular disease, diabetes, respiratory infections, pregnancy
complications, and dementia. Poor oral health, such as gum disease,
can contribute to inflammation throughout the body, which is a risk
factor for many chronic diseases.

2. Inflammation and Immune Response:

- Oral infections, such as gum disease, can trigger inflammatory
responses in the body, leading to systemic inflammation. Chronic
inflammation is associated with a wide range of health issues, including
heart disease, stroke, diabetes, and autoimmune disorders.

3. Oral Microbiome:

- The oral microbiome, which consists of bacteria, viruses, fungi, and
other microorganisms, plays a crucial role in maintaining oral health
and influencing overall health. Imbalances in the oral microbiome can
contribute to oral diseases such as tooth decay and gum disease, as
well as systemic health issues.

4. Gut-Brain Axis:

- The health of the mouth is closely connected to the gut microbiome
and the gut-brain axis, which influences digestive health, immune
function, and mental well-being. Imbalances in the oral microbiome
can impact gut health and contribute to gastrointestinal issues and
mental health disorders such as anxiety and depression.

5. Chronic Infections and Inflammatory Pathways:

- Chronic oral infections, such as untreated tooth decay or gum
disease, can serve as a source of chronic inflammation and infection in
the body. This can activate inflammatory pathways and increase the
risk of developing chronic diseases such as heart disease, diabetes, and
rheumatoid arthritis.

6. Impact on Nutrition and Diet:

- Oral health can influence nutrition and diet choices, as individuals with oral health issues may have difficulty chewing, swallowing, or tasting food. Poor oral health can also affect dietary intake and nutritional status, leading to deficiencies in essential nutrients that are important for overall health and well-being.

7. Psychosocial Impact:
  - Oral health can have a significant psychosocial impact on an individual's quality of life, self-esteem, and social interactions. Oral health issues such as missing teeth, dental pain, or bad breath can affect self-confidence, social relationships, and overall mental health and well-being.

8. Preventive Measures and Self-Care:
  - Maintaining good oral hygiene practices, such as brushing and flossing regularly, visiting the dentist for routine check-ups and cleanings, and adopting a healthy lifestyle, can help prevent oral health problems and reduce the risk of systemic health issues. Self-care practices that support oral health, such as eating a balanced diet, staying hydrated, avoiding tobacco use, and managing stress, are also essential for overall well-being.

Minimally Invasive Dental Practices

Minimally invasive dental practices are an integral component of holistic dentistry, emphasizing the preservation of natural tooth structure, patient comfort, and overall health and well-being. These practices focus on preventing dental problems, treating issues at the earliest stages, and using conservative treatment approaches whenever possible. Here are some key aspects of minimally invasive dental practices:

1. Preventive Care:
  - Preventive care is the foundation of minimally invasive dentistry and holistic oral health. It includes regular dental check-ups, professional cleanings, oral health education, and personalized preventive measures to maintain optimal oral health and prevent dental problems before they occur. By promoting good oral hygiene

habits and identifying risk factors early, preventive care helps reduce the need for invasive dental treatments.

2. **Early Intervention:**
- Minimally invasive dentistry focuses on early intervention and conservative treatment approaches to address dental issues at the earliest stages. This may involve detecting and treating cavities in their initial stages with techniques such as remineralization, fluoride therapy, and minimally invasive restorations such as dental sealants or composite resin fillings. By addressing dental problems promptly, before they progress, minimally invasive dentistry helps preserve natural tooth structure and avoid more extensive treatments.

3. **Preservation of Natural Tooth Structure:**
- Minimally invasive dental practices prioritize the preservation of natural tooth structure whenever possible. This includes techniques such as tooth-colored fillings, which bond to the tooth structure and require less removal of healthy tooth material compared to traditional amalgam fillings. Minimally invasive approaches aim to conserve as much healthy tooth structure as possible while effectively treating dental issues.

4. **Digital Dentistry:**
- Digital dentistry technologies, such as intraoral scanners, computer-aided design and manufacturing (CAD/CAM), and 3D imaging, enable dentists to plan and perform treatments with greater precision, efficiency, and minimal invasiveness. These technologies allow for more accurate diagnosis, treatment planning, and fabrication of restorations, reducing the need for invasive procedures and improving treatment outcomes.

5. **Laser Dentistry:**
- Laser dentistry utilizes advanced laser technology to perform a variety of dental procedures with minimal discomfort, bleeding, and recovery time. Lasers can be used for procedures such as cavity detection, gum disease treatment, gum contouring, and soft tissue surgeries. Laser dentistry is often less invasive than traditional techniques, as it can target specific areas with precision while preserving surrounding healthy tissue.

6. Biocompatible Materials:

   - Minimally invasive dentistry emphasizes the use of biocompatible dental materials that are safe for the body and minimize the risk of adverse reactions or sensitivities. This includes tooth-colored composite resins, porcelain restorations, and metal-free alternatives to traditional dental materials such as dental amalgam. Biocompatible materials support the body's natural healing processes and promote long-term oral health and well-being.

7. Patient-Centered Care:

   - Minimally invasive dentistry is patient-centered, focusing on the individual needs, preferences, and priorities of each patient. Dentists take the time to educate patients about their treatment options, involve them in decision-making processes, and address any concerns or questions they may have. By empowering patients to make informed decisions about their oral health care, minimally invasive dentistry promotes collaboration and trust between patients and providers.

Natural Approaches to Dental Care

Natural approaches to dental care encompass a range of holistic practices and strategies that prioritize the use of natural remedies, preventive measures, and lifestyle interventions to support optimal oral health and overall well-being. Here are some key aspects of natural approaches to dental care:

1. Nutrition and Diet:

   - A balanced diet rich in essential nutrients is essential for maintaining healthy teeth and gums. Nutrients such as calcium, vitamin D, vitamin C, and phosphorus are crucial for strong teeth and supporting oral health. Emphasizing whole foods such as fruits, vegetables, lean proteins, and dairy products, and minimizing the consumption of sugary and acidic foods can help prevent tooth decay and gum disease.

2. Hygiene Practices:

- Natural dental hygiene practices focus on gentle and effective methods for cleaning teeth and gums without the use of harsh chemicals or abrasive ingredients. This includes brushing teeth with fluoride-free toothpaste made from natural ingredients such as baking soda, coconut oil, and essential oils. Additionally, natural dental floss, mouthwash, and tongue cleaners can complement daily oral hygiene routines.

3. Oil Pulling:

- Oil pulling is an ancient Ayurvedic practice that involves swishing oil (such as coconut oil or sesame oil) in the mouth for several minutes to remove toxins, bacteria, and plaque from the teeth and gums. Oil pulling is believed to support oral health by reducing inflammation, preventing cavities, and promoting fresh breath.

4. Herbal Remedies:

- Herbal remedies have been used for centuries to promote oral health and treat various dental issues. Herbs such as neem, clove, peppermint, and tea tree oil have antibacterial, anti-inflammatory, and analgesic properties that can help prevent tooth decay, reduce gum inflammation, and alleviate dental pain. Herbal mouthwashes, tooth powders, and poultices are natural alternatives to conventional dental products.

5. Homeopathy:

- Homeopathic remedies can be used to support oral health and address dental problems such as toothaches, gum disease, and oral infections. Homeopathic remedies are selected based on the individual's unique symptoms and constitutional profile and can help stimulate the body's self-healing mechanisms and restore balance to the oral cavity.

6. Hydrotherapy:

- Hydrotherapy involves using water-based treatments to promote oral health and hygiene. Techniques such as warm saltwater rinses, herbal mouthwashes, and oral irrigation devices can help cleanse the mouth, reduce inflammation, and promote healing of oral tissues. Hydrotherapy can be used as a natural complement to regular oral hygiene practices.

7. Stress Reduction:

   - Stress can have a significant impact on oral health by contributing to teeth grinding (bruxism), jaw clenching, and gum disease. Practicing stress reduction techniques such as mindfulness meditation, deep breathing exercises, yoga, and massage therapy can help relax the jaw muscles, reduce tension, and promote overall oral health and well-being.

8. Preventive Measures:

   - Natural approaches to dental care emphasize preventive measures such as regular dental check-ups, professional cleanings, dental sealants, and fluoride-free preventive treatments. These measures help detect and address dental issues early, prevent tooth decay and gum disease, and maintain optimal oral health throughout life.

Holistic Perspectives on Orthodontics and Cosmetic Dentistry

Holistic perspectives on orthodontics and cosmetic dentistry integrate traditional dental practices with holistic principles to promote not only aesthetic improvements but also overall health and well-being. These approaches prioritize the preservation of natural tooth structure, biocompatibility of materials, and consideration of systemic health implications. Here's an overview of holistic perspectives on orthodontics and cosmetic dentistry:

1. Preservation of Natural Tooth Structure:

   - Holistic orthodontics and cosmetic dentistry emphasize preserving as much natural tooth structure as possible while achieving desired aesthetic outcomes. Rather than focusing solely on straightening teeth or enhancing appearance, these approaches prioritize the health and integrity of the teeth and surrounding tissues. Minimally invasive techniques, such as clear aligners and tooth-colored braces, may be preferred to traditional orthodontic treatments that require significant enamel removal or alteration.

2. Biocompatibility of Materials:

- Holistic practitioners prioritize the use of biocompatible materials in orthodontic and cosmetic treatments to minimize potential adverse reactions or sensitivities. This includes avoiding materials such as metal alloys containing nickel or mercury-based dental materials, which may pose risks to systemic health and overall well-being. Instead, biocompatible alternatives such as ceramic, composite resin, or porcelain materials may be used for orthodontic appliances, dental crowns, veneers, and other cosmetic restorations.

3. Systemic Health Considerations:

- Holistic orthodontics and cosmetic dentistry take into account the systemic health implications of dental treatments and their potential impact on overall well-being. For example, orthodontic treatments that improve dental alignment can also support proper jaw function, bite alignment, and airway patency, which are important factors for respiratory health, sleep quality, and overall systemic function. By addressing underlying structural issues and promoting optimal oral function, holistic approaches to orthodontics and cosmetic dentistry can contribute to improved overall health and well-being.

4. Functional and Aesthetic Balance:

- Holistic practitioners strive to achieve a balance between functional improvements and aesthetic enhancements in orthodontic and cosmetic treatments. This involves considering not only the appearance of the teeth and smile but also their function, alignment, and relationship to the jaw and surrounding structures. By optimizing both functional and aesthetic aspects of oral health, holistic approaches seek to create harmonious and balanced outcomes that support overall health and well-being.

5. Individualized Treatment Plans:

- Holistic orthodontics and cosmetic dentistry recognize that each patient is unique and may have different needs, preferences, and health considerations. Treatment plans are personalized to address the individual's specific concerns and goals while taking into account their overall health status, lifestyle factors, and holistic principles. This may involve a combination of orthodontic, cosmetic, and preventive measures tailored to the patient's needs and circumstances.

6. Collaborative Care:

- Holistic orthodontics and cosmetic dentistry involve collaboration between dental professionals and other healthcare providers to provide comprehensive care that addresses the patient's overall health and well-being. This may include working with functional medicine practitioners, osteopaths, chiropractors, physical therapists, and other healthcare professionals to address underlying systemic issues, optimize oral function, and promote holistic healing.

Chapter 8
Holistic Approaches
to Sleep

The Importance of Quality Sleep in Holistic Health

Quality sleep is a cornerstone of holistic health, essential for supporting physical, mental, and emotional well-being. Holistic approaches to sleep recognize the interconnectedness of sleep with other aspects of health and emphasize the importance of achieving restorative sleep for overall vitality. Here's why quality sleep is crucial in holistic health:

1. Physical Restoration:
- During sleep, the body undergoes essential processes of repair, regeneration, and restoration. This includes the repair of tissues and muscles, the consolidation of memories, the release of growth hormones, and the regulation of metabolic functions. Quality sleep is necessary to support these physiological processes and promote optimal physical health and vitality.

2. Immune Function:
- Adequate sleep plays a vital role in supporting a robust immune system. Sleep deprivation has been shown to weaken immune function, increasing the risk of infections, inflammation, and chronic diseases. Quality sleep helps regulate immune responses, enhances immune cell activity, and strengthens the body's defenses against pathogens and illnesses.

3. Mental Clarity and Cognitive Function:
- Sleep is essential for cognitive function, learning, memory consolidation, and emotional regulation. Quality sleep improves concentration, focus, problem-solving abilities, and decision-making skills. Chronic sleep deprivation, on the other hand, can impair cognitive performance, memory retention, and emotional resilience, leading to decreased productivity, mood disturbances, and mental health issues.

4. Emotional Well-Being:
- Sleep plays a crucial role in regulating emotions and maintaining emotional well-being. Adequate sleep supports mood stability, stress resilience, and psychological resilience. Sleep deprivation, on the other hand, is associated with increased irritability, mood swings, anxiety,

depression, and other mental health disorders. Quality sleep promotes emotional balance, enhances coping mechanisms, and fosters a positive outlook on life.

5. Hormonal Balance:
- Sleep is intricately linked to hormonal balance, including hormones that regulate appetite, metabolism, stress responses, and reproductive function. Quality sleep helps maintain hormonal equilibrium, supporting healthy weight management, stress resilience, and reproductive health. Chronic sleep disturbances disrupt hormonal balance, contributing to weight gain, hormonal imbalances, and metabolic disorders.

6. Regulation of Circadian Rhythms:
- Sleep plays a crucial role in regulating circadian rhythms, the body's internal clock that governs various physiological processes, including sleep-wake cycles, hormone secretion, body temperature, and metabolism. Quality sleep at regular times helps synchronize circadian rhythms, promoting overall health, vitality, and longevity. Disruptions to circadian rhythms, such as shift work or irregular sleep patterns, can negatively impact health and increase the risk of chronic diseases.

7. Stress Reduction and Resilience:
- Quality sleep is essential for stress reduction and resilience. During sleep, the body relaxes, and stress hormones such as cortisol decrease, allowing for physical and emotional recovery. Adequate sleep enhances stress resilience, improves coping mechanisms, and reduces the risk of burnout, anxiety, and depression. Chronic sleep deprivation, on the other hand, can increase stress levels, exacerbate stress-related symptoms, and impair overall well-being.

Sleep Hygiene Practices

Sleep hygiene practices are fundamental to achieving restful and rejuvenating sleep. They encompass a set of behaviors and habits that promote optimal sleep quality and quantity. Incorporating these practices into your daily routine can help improve sleep patterns and enhance overall well-being. Here are some essential sleep hygiene practices:

1. Maintain a Consistent Sleep Schedule:

- Go to bed and wake up at the same time every day, even on weekends. Consistency helps regulate your body's internal clock and promote better sleep quality.

2. Create a Relaxing Bedtime Routine:

- Establish a calming pre-sleep routine to signal to your body that it's time to wind down. This may include activities such as reading, taking a warm bath, practicing relaxation techniques like deep breathing or meditation, or listening to soothing music.

3. Create a Comfortable Sleep Environment:

- Make your bedroom conducive to sleep by keeping it dark, quiet, cool, and comfortable. Consider using blackout curtains, earplugs, white noise machines, or a comfortable mattress and pillows to optimize your sleep environment.

4. Limit Exposure to Screens Before Bed:

- Reduce exposure to electronic devices such as smartphones, tablets, computers, and TVs at least an hour before bedtime. The blue light emitted by screens can suppress melatonin production and disrupt your sleep-wake cycle.

5. Mindful Eating and Drinking:

- Avoid heavy meals, caffeine, nicotine, and alcohol close to bedtime, as they can interfere with your ability to fall asleep and stay asleep. Instead, opt for light, easily digestible snacks if you're hungry, and limit caffeine and alcohol consumption earlier in the day.

6. Get Regular Exercise:

- Engage in regular physical activity during the day, but avoid vigorous exercise close to bedtime, as it can be stimulating and interfere with your ability to relax and fall asleep. Aim for moderate-intensity exercise earlier in the day to promote better sleep.

7. Manage Stress and Anxiety:

- Practice stress-reduction techniques such as mindfulness meditation, progressive muscle relaxation, or journaling to help calm your mind and alleviate anxiety before bedtime. If you find yourself worrying or ruminating, try writing down your thoughts or making a to-do list for the next day to clear your mind.

8. Limit Naps During the Day:
- While short naps can be beneficial for some people, particularly if they're feeling tired or sleep-deprived, avoid long or late-afternoon naps, as they can disrupt your nighttime sleep patterns. If you need to nap, aim for a brief nap of 20-30 minutes earlier in the day to avoid interfering with nighttime sleep.

9. Seek Natural Light Exposure:
- Get exposure to natural sunlight during the day, especially in the morning. Natural light helps regulate your body's circadian rhythm and promote wakefulness during the day, which can improve sleep quality and daytime alertness.

10. Limit Stimulating Activities in Bed:
- Reserve your bed for sleep and intimacy. Avoid engaging in stimulating activities such as working, watching TV, or using electronic devices in bed, as they can associate your bed with wakefulness rather than relaxation.

Mind-Body Techniques for Better Sleep

Mind-body techniques are valuable tools for improving sleep quality by addressing both the mental and physical aspects of sleep. These practices promote relaxation, reduce stress, and enhance overall well-being, making them effective for achieving restful and rejuvenating sleep. Here are some mind-body techniques that can help improve sleep:

1. Progressive Muscle Relaxation (PMR):
- PMR involves systematically tensing and relaxing different muscle groups throughout the body to release tension and promote relaxation. Start by tensing each muscle group for a few seconds and then

gradually releasing the tension while focusing on the sensation of relaxation. This technique can help alleviate physical tension and prepare the body for sleep.

2. Deep Breathing Exercises:

   - Deep breathing exercises, such as diaphragmatic breathing or belly breathing, involve taking slow, deep breaths to activate the body's relaxation response. Focus on breathing deeply into your diaphragm, allowing your belly to rise and fall with each breath. Deep breathing can help calm the mind, reduce stress, and promote feelings of relaxation conducive to sleep.

3. Mindfulness Meditation:

   - Mindfulness meditation involves paying attention to the present moment with openness, curiosity, and acceptance, without judgment. By practicing mindfulness meditation before bedtime, you can cultivate a sense of calmness and presence, quiet the mind, and let go of racing thoughts or worries that may interfere with sleep. Guided mindfulness meditation recordings or apps can be helpful for beginners.

4. Yoga and Gentle Stretching:

   - Gentle yoga poses and stretching exercises can help release tension from the body, promote relaxation, and prepare the body for sleep. Focus on gentle, restorative yoga poses that emphasize deep breathing and relaxation, such as child's pose, forward bends, and gentle twists. Yoga nidra, or yogic sleep, is a guided meditation practice that combines relaxation techniques with mindfulness and can be particularly effective for promoting sleep.

5. Visualization and Imagery:

   - Visualization and imagery techniques involve mentally picturing calming scenes or peaceful images to promote relaxation and induce sleep. Close your eyes and imagine yourself in a tranquil setting, such as a beach, forest, or meadow, focusing on the sights, sounds, and sensations of the environment. Visualization can help quiet the mind and create a sense of serenity conducive to sleep.

6. Aromatherapy:

- Aromatherapy involves using essential oils to promote relaxation and improve sleep quality. Lavender, chamomile, and bergamot are among the essential oils known for their calming and sleep-inducing properties. Diffuse these oils in your bedroom, add a few drops to a warm bath, or apply them to your skin using a carrier oil before bedtime to promote relaxation and enhance sleep.

7. Biofeedback and Relaxation Techniques:

- Biofeedback techniques involve using electronic devices to monitor and control physiological responses such as heart rate, muscle tension, and skin temperature. Biofeedback can help increase awareness of bodily sensations and teach individuals to consciously regulate their physiological responses, promoting relaxation and stress reduction conducive to sleep.

8. Cognitive Behavioral Therapy for Insomnia (CBT-I):

- CBT-I is a structured, evidence-based therapy that addresses dysfunctional thoughts and behaviors related to sleep. It helps individuals identify and challenge negative thought patterns, establish healthy sleep habits, and develop relaxation techniques to improve sleep quality and quantity. CBT-I has been shown to be highly effective for treating insomnia and promoting better sleep.

Herbal and Natural Remedies for Sleep

Herbal and natural remedies offer gentle and holistic approaches to promoting better sleep without the potential side effects associated with pharmaceutical sleep aids. These remedies work synergistically with the body's natural processes to calm the mind, relax the body, and induce restful sleep. Here are some herbal and natural remedies that can help improve sleep quality:

1. Valerian Root:

- Valerian root is a popular herb known for its calming and sedative properties. It contains compounds that act on the nervous system to promote relaxation and improve sleep quality. Valerian root can be consumed as a tea, tincture, or supplement, typically taken 30 minutes to an hour before bedtime.

2. Chamomile:

- Chamomile is a gentle herb with soothing and calming properties. It contains compounds such as apigenin that promote relaxation and reduce anxiety, making it an excellent choice for promoting sleep. Chamomile tea is a popular and effective natural remedy for sleep and can be consumed in the evening to help unwind and prepare for bedtime.

3. Lavender:

- Lavender is renowned for its calming and aromatic properties, which can help promote relaxation and improve sleep quality. Inhalation of lavender essential oil or using lavender sachets in your bedroom can create a soothing environment conducive to sleep. Additionally, lavender tea or lavender-infused bath products can help promote relaxation before bedtime.

4. Passionflower:

- Passionflower is a gentle herb with sedative properties that can help calm the mind and promote restful sleep. It contains compounds that increase levels of gamma-aminobutyric acid (GABA), a neurotransmitter that promotes relaxation and reduces anxiety. Passionflower tea or supplements can be consumed before bedtime to help improve sleep quality.

5. Lemon Balm:

- Lemon balm is a member of the mint family known for its calming and mood-enhancing effects. It contains compounds that promote relaxation and reduce stress and anxiety, making it beneficial for improving sleep quality. Lemon balm tea or supplements can be consumed in the evening to help promote relaxation and prepare for sleep.

6. Ashwagandha:

- Ashwagandha is an adaptogenic herb that helps the body adapt to stress and promotes relaxation. It can help reduce cortisol levels, calm the mind, and improve sleep quality. Ashwagandha supplements or powdered root can be consumed in the evening to help manage stress and promote better sleep.

7. **Magnesium:**
   - Magnesium is an essential mineral that plays a key role in relaxation and sleep regulation. Magnesium deficiency has been linked to sleep disturbances and insomnia. Consuming magnesium-rich foods such as leafy greens, nuts, seeds, and whole grains, or taking a magnesium supplement before bedtime, can help promote relaxation and improve sleep quality.

8. **Melatonin:**
   - Melatonin is a hormone naturally produced by the body that regulates the sleep-wake cycle. Supplemental melatonin can be used to help reset the body's internal clock and improve sleep quality, particularly for individuals with sleep disorders or jet lag. Melatonin supplements should be taken as directed, typically 30 minutes to an hour before bedtime.

Before using herbal or natural remedies for sleep, it's essential to consult with a healthcare professional, especially if you have underlying health conditions or are taking medications. While herbal remedies are generally considered safe, they may interact with certain medications or have contraindications for certain individuals. Additionally, incorporating relaxation techniques, establishing a consistent sleep routine, and creating a comfortable sleep environment are important components of holistic sleep hygiene practices that can complement the use of herbal and natural remedies for better sleep.

Addressing Sleep Disorders Holistically

Addressing sleep disorders holistically involves identifying and addressing the underlying causes of sleep disturbances while promoting overall health and well-being. Holistic approaches to sleep disorders recognize the interconnectedness of physical, mental, and emotional factors that contribute to sleep disturbances and aim to restore balance and promote restful sleep naturally. Here are some holistic strategies for addressing sleep disorders:

1. **Identify Underlying Causes:**

- Holistic practitioners take a comprehensive approach to identify
and address the underlying causes of sleep disorders. This may involve
evaluating lifestyle factors, stress levels, dietary habits, hormonal
imbalances, medical conditions, medication side effects, and
environmental factors that may be contributing to sleep disturbances.
By addressing the root causes of sleep disorders, holistic approaches
focus on promoting long-term improvements in sleep quality and
overall health.

2. Optimize Sleep Hygiene:

- Sleep hygiene practices form the foundation of holistic sleep
management. Individuals are encouraged to adopt healthy sleep habits
such as maintaining a consistent sleep schedule, creating a relaxing
bedtime routine, creating a comfortable sleep environment, limiting
screen time before bed, and avoiding stimulants such as caffeine and
alcohol close to bedtime. By optimizing sleep hygiene, individuals can
improve their sleep quality and quantity naturally.

3. Manage Stress and Anxiety:

- Stress and anxiety are common contributors to sleep disorders such
as insomnia. Holistic approaches emphasize stress reduction techniques
such as mindfulness meditation, deep breathing exercises, yoga,
progressive muscle relaxation, and cognitive-behavioral therapy (CBT)
to promote relaxation and alleviate anxiety before bedtime. By
managing stress and anxiety, individuals can create a more conducive
environment for restful sleep.

4. Promote Relaxation and Mind-Body Balance:

- Holistic modalities such as acupuncture, acupressure, massage
therapy, aromatherapy, and biofeedback can help promote relaxation,
reduce tension, and restore balance to the body's energy systems.
These practices can help alleviate physical discomfort, promote
relaxation, and enhance overall well-being, contributing to improved
sleep quality and sleep disorders management.

5. Nutritional Support:

- Nutrition plays a crucial role in sleep health, and holistic
approaches may include dietary modifications to support better sleep.
Incorporating nutrient-rich foods such as fruits, vegetables, whole

grains, lean proteins, and healthy fats into the diet can help regulate sleep-wake cycles and promote relaxation. Avoiding heavy meals, caffeine, and alcohol close to bedtime can also improve sleep quality.

6. Herbal and Natural Remedies:
   - Herbal and natural remedies such as valerian root, chamomile, passionflower, lavender, and melatonin may be used to support better sleep naturally. These remedies have calming and sedative properties that can help promote relaxation, reduce anxiety, and improve sleep quality without the side effects associated with pharmaceutical sleep aids. However, it's essential to consult with a healthcare professional before using herbal remedies, especially if you have underlying health conditions or are taking medications.

7. Address Sleep Environment and Lifestyle Factors:
   - Holistic approaches involve evaluating and addressing environmental factors that may disrupt sleep, such as noise, light, temperature, and comfort. Making adjustments to create a sleep-friendly environment can help improve sleep quality. Additionally, adopting a healthy lifestyle that includes regular exercise, a balanced diet, stress management, and social support can contribute to better overall sleep health.

8. Seek Professional Guidance:
   - If sleep disturbances persist despite holistic interventions, it's essential to seek professional guidance from a healthcare provider or sleep specialist. They can help diagnose and treat underlying sleep disorders, provide personalized recommendations, and offer additional treatment options such as cognitive-behavioral therapy for insomnia (CBT-I) or sleep studies to assess sleep disorders more comprehensively.

Chapter 9 Environmental Wellness

Holistic Perspectives on Environmental Health

Holistic perspectives on environmental health emphasize the interconnectedness between the health of individuals and the health of the environment. These perspectives recognize that environmental factors play a significant role in shaping human health and well-being and advocate for sustainable practices that support both human health and the health of the planet. Here are some key principles of holistic perspectives on environmental health:

1. **Interconnectedness of Humans and the Environment:**
   - Holistic perspectives view humans as integral parts of the environment, deeply interconnected with the natural world. Environmental health is not seen as separate from human health but rather as intertwined systems that influence each other. The quality of the air we breathe, the water we drink, the food we eat, and the places we live and work directly impacts our health and well-being.

2. **Prevention and Precaution:**
   - Holistic approaches to environmental health prioritize prevention and precautionary principles to minimize harm and protect human and environmental health. Instead of reacting to health problems after they arise, these approaches focus on identifying and addressing potential hazards before they become significant threats. This involves assessing risks, adopting proactive measures, and promoting sustainable practices that prevent environmental degradation and promote health and well-being.

3. **Whole Systems Thinking:**
   - Holistic perspectives on environmental health embrace whole systems thinking, recognizing the complex interactions and interdependencies between various environmental factors and human health outcomes. Rather than addressing environmental issues in isolation, these approaches consider the broader ecological context and seek holistic solutions that address underlying systemic causes and promote synergistic benefits for both human health and environmental sustainability.

4. **Promotion of Ecological Balance:**

- Holistic approaches prioritize the preservation and restoration of ecological balance and biodiversity as essential components of environmental health. Healthy ecosystems provide essential services such as clean air, clean water, fertile soil, pollination, and climate regulation, which are critical for supporting human health and well-being. Protecting and restoring natural habitats, conserving biodiversity, and promoting sustainable land management practices are central to holistic environmental health strategies.

5. Prevention of Pollution and Contamination:

- Holistic perspectives advocate for minimizing pollution and contamination of air, water, soil, and food sources to safeguard human and environmental health. This involves reducing emissions of toxic pollutants, minimizing exposure to harmful chemicals and pollutants, and promoting cleaner, more sustainable alternatives in industrial processes, agriculture, transportation, and energy production.

6. Promotion of Sustainable Practices:

- Holistic approaches to environmental health promote sustainable practices that support ecological integrity, social equity, and economic viability. This includes reducing resource consumption, minimizing waste generation, promoting renewable energy sources, supporting local and organic food systems, and fostering resilient communities that prioritize health, equity, and environmental stewardship.

7. Community Engagement and Empowerment:

- Holistic environmental health strategies prioritize community engagement, participation, and empowerment, recognizing that individuals and communities have valuable knowledge, experiences, and resources that can contribute to environmental protection and health promotion. Empowering communities to participate in decision-making processes, advocate for their rights, and implement locally appropriate solutions fosters a sense of ownership, resilience, and collective action towards shared environmental and health goals.

Creating a Healthy Home Environment

Creating a healthy home environment is essential for promoting overall well-being and supporting holistic health. Our homes are where we spend a significant amount of time, and the indoor environment can have a profound impact on our physical, mental, and emotional health. Here are some holistic strategies for creating a healthy home environment:

1. **Ensure Clean Air Quality:**
  - Indoor air quality can significantly affect respiratory health and overall well-being. To improve air quality:
    - Use natural cleaning products and avoid harsh chemicals, which can release volatile organic compounds (VOCs) and other pollutants into the air.
    - Keep indoor plants, which can help purify the air by absorbing pollutants and releasing oxygen.
    - Install high-efficiency particulate air (HEPA) filters in HVAC systems to remove airborne particles, allergens, and pollutants.
    - Ventilate your home regularly by opening windows and using exhaust fans, especially when cooking or using cleaning products.

2. **Reduce Exposure to Toxic Substances:**
  - Minimize exposure to harmful chemicals and toxins found in household products, building materials, furniture, and electronics. Choose natural, non-toxic alternatives whenever possible, and look for products labeled as eco-friendly, organic, or low-VOC.
  - Avoid synthetic fragrances, which can contain phthalates and other harmful chemicals. Opt for fragrance-free or naturally scented products instead.
  - Test your home for radon, a naturally occurring radioactive gas that can seep into buildings from the ground. Radon testing kits are available for purchase, and mitigation measures can be taken if elevated levels are detected.

3. **Promote Water Quality and Safety:**
  - Ensure that your drinking water is clean and safe by testing it regularly for contaminants such as lead, bacteria, and chemicals. Consider installing a water filtration system to remove impurities and improve taste.

- Avoid using plastic water bottles, which can leach harmful chemicals such as bisphenol A (BPA) and phthalates into the water. Opt for reusable glass or stainless steel water bottles instead.

4. Create a Restful Sleep Environment:
- Design your bedroom to promote restful sleep and relaxation:
- Choose a comfortable mattress and pillows that provide adequate support.
- Keep the bedroom dark, quiet, and cool to create an optimal sleep environment.
- Limit exposure to electronic devices such as smartphones, computers, and TVs before bedtime, as the blue light emitted can disrupt sleep-wake cycles.

5. Support Emotional Well-Being:
- Create a nurturing and supportive environment that fosters emotional well-being:
- Incorporate elements of nature into your home decor, such as plants, natural materials, and sunlight, which can promote feelings of calmness and connection to the natural world.
- Designate spaces for relaxation, meditation, and mindfulness practice, such as a cozy reading nook or a meditation corner.
- Foster positive social connections by creating inviting spaces for gatherings and fostering open communication with family members and housemates.

6. Maintain a Clutter-Free Environment:
- Clutter can contribute to stress, anxiety, and feelings of overwhelm. Keep your home organized and clutter-free by regularly decluttering and organizing belongings. Simplify your living space by prioritizing items that bring you joy and purpose, and consider donating or recycling items that you no longer need or use.

7. Promote Sustainable Living Practices:
- Adopt eco-friendly practices that reduce your environmental footprint and support sustainability:
- Reduce energy consumption by using energy-efficient appliances, LED light bulbs, and programmable thermostats.

- Conserve water by fixing leaks, installing low-flow fixtures, and practicing water-saving habits such as taking shorter showers and using water-efficient landscaping.
- Reduce waste by recycling, composting organic materials, and minimizing single-use plastics and packaging.

Navigating Environmental Toxins

Navigating environmental toxins is essential for promoting environmental wellness and supporting holistic health. In today's world, we are exposed to various pollutants and toxins in our environment, including air and water pollutants, chemicals in household products, pesticides in food, and contaminants in everyday items. Here are some holistic strategies for navigating environmental toxins:

1. **Education and Awareness:**
   - Educate yourself about common environmental toxins and their potential health effects. Stay informed about emerging research and recommendations from reputable sources such as environmental agencies, health organizations, and scientific publications.
   - Be aware of sources of environmental toxins in your daily life, including air pollution, water contamination, household chemicals, personal care products, food additives, and industrial pollutants.

2. **Reduce Exposure:**
   - Minimize your exposure to environmental toxins by making conscious choices to reduce or eliminate sources of pollution and contamination:
   - Choose organic produce whenever possible to reduce exposure to pesticides and herbicides.
   - Opt for natural, non-toxic household cleaning products and personal care items, and avoid products containing harmful chemicals such as phthalates, parabens, sulfates, and synthetic fragrances.
   - Filter your drinking water to remove contaminants such as lead, chlorine, fluoride, and industrial pollutants.
   - Ventilate your home to reduce indoor air pollution, and avoid exposure to tobacco smoke, radon gas, and other indoor pollutants.

- Be cautious when using plastics, especially those containing bisphenol A (BPA) and phthalates, which can leach into food and beverages. Choose glass, stainless steel, or BPA-free plastics for food storage and beverage containers.
- Use natural pest control methods in your home and garden, and avoid the use of chemical pesticides and insecticides.

3. Support Detoxification:
- Support your body's natural detoxification processes to help eliminate toxins and pollutants:
- Stay hydrated by drinking plenty of clean, filtered water to support kidney function and flush out toxins.
- Eat a healthy, balanced diet rich in fruits, vegetables, whole grains, and lean proteins, which provide essential nutrients and antioxidants that support detoxification.
- Incorporate foods that support liver health, such as cruciferous vegetables (broccoli, cabbage, kale), garlic, onions, turmeric, and green tea.
- Engage in regular physical activity, which promotes circulation, lymphatic drainage, and sweating, all of which help eliminate toxins from the body.
- Consider incorporating detoxifying practices such as sauna therapy, dry brushing, lymphatic massage, and herbal supplements that support liver and kidney function.

4. Promote Environmental Stewardship:
- Advocate for policies and practices that protect the environment and reduce exposure to toxins on a broader scale:
- Support regulations and initiatives aimed at reducing air and water pollution, limiting industrial emissions, and promoting clean energy and sustainable agriculture.
- Participate in community efforts to clean up pollution, conserve natural resources, and promote environmental justice and equity.
- Reduce waste and pollution by recycling, composting, and minimizing consumption of single-use plastics and disposable products.
- Support companies and brands that prioritize environmental sustainability, transparency, and ethical sourcing practices.

5. Practice Mindfulness and Stress Reduction:

- Chronic stress can weaken the immune system and exacerbate the effects of environmental toxins on health. Practice mindfulness, stress reduction techniques, and self-care practices to promote resilience and support overall well-being:
    - Practice deep breathing exercises, meditation, yoga, tai chi, or other relaxation techniques to reduce stress and promote mental clarity.
    - Spend time in nature, engage in creative activities, and cultivate positive social connections to foster a sense of peace, joy, and connection with the natural world.
    - Limit exposure to negative news and media, and focus on activities and experiences that bring you joy, fulfillment, and a sense of purpose.

Sustainable Living Practices

Sustainable living practices are integral to environmental wellness and promote harmony between individuals and the natural world. These practices prioritize the responsible use of resources, minimize environmental impact, and support long-term ecological balance. By adopting sustainable living practices, individuals can reduce their ecological footprint, conserve natural resources, and promote environmental health and well-being. Here are some holistic strategies for incorporating sustainable living practices into daily life:

1. **Reduce Energy Consumption:**
    - Conserve energy by implementing energy-efficient practices in your home and daily routines:
    - Use energy-efficient appliances and lighting, such as LED bulbs, ENERGY STAR-rated appliances, and programmable thermostats.
    - Turn off lights, electronics, and appliances when not in use, and unplug chargers and devices to reduce standby power consumption.
    - Seal drafts and insulate your home to improve energy efficiency and reduce heating and cooling costs.
    - Opt for renewable energy sources such as solar panels or wind turbines to generate clean, renewable electricity for your home.

2. **Conserve Water:**

- Practice water conservation to protect this vital resource and reduce water usage:
   - Fix leaks, drips, and plumbing issues promptly to prevent water waste.
   - Install water-saving fixtures such as low-flow toilets, showerheads, and faucets to reduce water consumption.
   - Collect rainwater for outdoor irrigation and landscaping, and use drought-tolerant plants in your garden to minimize water usage.
   - Limit water usage during daily activities such as bathing, washing dishes, and doing laundry, and consider using graywater systems to recycle water for non-potable purposes.

3. Minimize Waste:
   - Reduce waste generation and promote recycling, composting, and waste reduction practices:
   - Reduce single-use plastics and disposable items by opting for reusable alternatives such as stainless steel water bottles, cloth shopping bags, and reusable food containers.
   - Recycle paper, glass, metal, and plastic materials whenever possible, and support recycling programs in your community.
   - Compost organic waste such as food scraps, yard trimmings, and paper products to divert waste from landfills and create nutrient-rich soil for gardening.
   - Practice mindful consumption and reduce unnecessary packaging, disposable products, and items that contribute to landfill waste.

4. Promote Sustainable Transportation:
   - Reduce carbon emissions and air pollution by choosing sustainable transportation options:
   - Walk, bike, or use public transportation whenever possible to reduce reliance on fossil fuel-powered vehicles and promote physical activity.
   - Carpool or rideshare with others to reduce traffic congestion and vehicle emissions, and consider investing in fuel-efficient or electric vehicles for longer journeys.
   - Combine errands and trips to minimize vehicle miles traveled, and plan routes to optimize fuel efficiency and reduce travel time.

5. Support Sustainable Food Systems:

- Make informed choices about food consumption and support
sustainable food production practices:
    - Choose locally grown, seasonal, and organic foods whenever
possible to support local farmers, reduce transportation emissions, and
promote biodiversity.
    - Minimize food waste by planning meals, storing food properly, and
composting leftover scraps.
    - Reduce consumption of animal products and prioritize plant-based
foods to lower greenhouse gas emissions, conserve water, and promote
animal welfare.
    - Grow your own fruits, vegetables, and herbs at home using organic
gardening practices, or participate in community-supported agriculture
(CSA) programs to access fresh, locally grown produce.

6. **Promote Environmental Stewardship:**
    - Advocate for policies and practices that promote environmental
conservation, sustainability, and social equity:
    - Support initiatives to protect natural habitats, conserve
biodiversity, and restore ecosystems through reforestation, habitat
restoration, and conservation efforts.
    - Participate in community clean-up events, tree planting activities,
and environmental education programs to raise awareness and promote
positive environmental action.
    - Vote for political leaders and policies that prioritize environmental
protection, renewable energy, and sustainable development at the
local, national, and global levels.
    - Engage in advocacy and activism to address environmental
injustices, promote environmental justice, and support marginalized
communities disproportionately affected by environmental hazards and
pollution.

Holistic Approaches to Outdoor and Indoor Spaces

Holistic approaches to outdoor and indoor spaces emphasize creating
environments that support overall well-being and promote harmony
between individuals and their surroundings. These approaches
recognize the interconnectedness between the built environment,
natural world, and human health, and aim to design spaces that

enhance physical, mental, and emotional well-being. Here are some holistic strategies for creating healthy and harmonious outdoor and indoor spaces:

Outdoor Spaces:

1. **Connect with Nature:**
   - Design outdoor spaces that promote connection with the natural world, such as gardens, green spaces, parks, and nature trails. Incorporate elements such as plants, trees, water features, and natural materials to create a sense of tranquility, vitality, and connection to nature.

2. **Promote Physical Activity:**
   - Design outdoor spaces that encourage physical activity and movement, such as walking paths, bike lanes, playgrounds, and sports facilities. Create opportunities for recreation, exercise, and outdoor activities that support physical health and well-being.

3. **Support Biodiversity:**
   - Create outdoor environments that support biodiversity and ecological balance by preserving natural habitats, planting native species, and providing food and shelter for wildlife. Design landscapes that promote pollination, soil health, and natural pest control to enhance ecological resilience and promote environmental health.

4. **Enhance Environmental Quality:**
   - Design outdoor spaces with consideration for environmental quality, such as air and water quality, noise pollution, and climate resilience. Incorporate green infrastructure, such as rain gardens, bioswales, and permeable surfaces, to manage stormwater runoff, improve air quality, and mitigate urban heat island effects.

5. **Provide Restorative Spaces:**
   - Design outdoor spaces that offer opportunities for relaxation, stress reduction, and restoration of mental and emotional well-being. Create quiet, peaceful areas with seating, shade, and natural elements that promote mindfulness, meditation, and connection with the natural world.

Indoor Spaces:

1. Maximize Natural Light and Ventilation:
- Design indoor spaces to maximize natural light and ventilation, which promote circadian rhythms, mood regulation, and overall health and well-being. Incorporate windows, skylights, and glass doors to bring in natural daylight and views of the outdoors. Use operable windows, vents, and fans to facilitate airflow and indoor air quality.

2. Create Healthy Indoor Environments:
- Design indoor spaces with consideration for indoor air quality, acoustics, lighting, and thermal comfort. Use non-toxic building materials, finishes, and furnishings to minimize off-gassing of volatile organic compounds (VOCs) and indoor air pollutants. Provide adequate ventilation, filtration, and humidity control to promote indoor air quality and occupant health.

3. Promote Biophilic Design:
- Incorporate biophilic design principles into indoor spaces to enhance connections with nature and support human health and well-being. Integrate natural elements such as plants, water features, natural materials, and views of nature into interior design to reduce stress, improve cognitive function, and foster a sense of well-being.

4. Design for Functionality and Flexibility:
- Design indoor spaces that support a variety of activities, functions, and user needs. Create flexible, adaptable spaces that can accommodate different uses, preferences, and lifestyles. Incorporate ergonomic design principles to promote comfort, efficiency, and productivity in indoor environments.

5. Promote Emotional Wellness and Comfort:
- Design indoor spaces that promote emotional wellness, comfort, and positive experiences. Consider factors such as lighting, color, texture, furniture layout, and sensory elements to create environments that feel welcoming, nurturing, and supportive of mental and emotional well-being.

6. Integrate Technology Mindfully:

   - Use technology mindfully and purposefully in indoor spaces to enhance comfort, convenience, and connectivity while minimizing potential negative impacts on health and well-being. Incorporate energy-efficient lighting, smart controls, and digital interfaces that promote user comfort, energy conservation, and environmental sustainability.

Chapter 10
Spiritual Well-Being

The Role of Spirituality in Holistic Health

Spirituality plays a vital role in holistic health, encompassing the interconnectedness of mind, body, and spirit. It involves seeking meaning, purpose, and connection to something greater than oneself and encompasses beliefs, values, practices, and experiences that foster a sense of inner peace, harmony, and transcendence. Here's how spirituality contributes to holistic health:

1. Meaning and Purpose:
   - Spirituality provides individuals with a sense of meaning and purpose in life, helping them understand their place in the world and navigate life's challenges with resilience and purpose. Beliefs and values rooted in spirituality guide individuals in making meaningful choices, setting goals, and finding fulfillment in their lives.

2. Connection and Belonging:
   - Spirituality fosters a sense of connection and belonging to oneself, others, and the universe. It promotes empathy, compassion, and interconnectedness with all living beings, fostering a sense of unity and shared humanity. Spiritual practices such as meditation, prayer, and mindfulness cultivate awareness and deepen connections with oneself, others, and the divine.

3. Inner Peace and Well-Being:
   - Spirituality offers a pathway to inner peace, tranquility, and well-being by nurturing a sense of harmony, acceptance, and surrender. Spiritual practices promote self-awareness, self-compassion, and self-transcendence, helping individuals navigate stress, anxiety, and emotional challenges with grace and equanimity.

4. Healing and Transformation:
   - Spirituality serves as a source of healing and transformation, addressing not only physical ailments but also emotional, psychological, and existential suffering. Spiritual practices such as meditation, yoga, and energy healing facilitate healing on multiple levels, supporting holistic well-being and promoting integration of mind, body, and spirit.

5. Resilience and Coping:

- Spirituality enhances resilience and coping skills, helping individuals navigate adversity, loss, and trauma with courage, faith, and hope. Spiritual beliefs and practices provide comfort, strength, and guidance during difficult times, offering solace, perspective, and a sense of transcendence beyond immediate challenges.

6. Health and Longevity:
- Research suggests that spirituality is associated with better health outcomes, increased longevity, and improved quality of life. Spiritual practices such as prayer, meditation, and mindfulness have been linked to reduced stress, improved immune function, lower blood pressure, and enhanced psychological well-being, contributing to overall health and vitality.

7. Integration of Mind, Body, and Spirit:
- Spirituality promotes the integration of mind, body, and spirit, recognizing the interconnectedness and interdependence of all aspects of human existence. Holistic health approaches emphasize the importance of addressing spiritual needs alongside physical, mental, and emotional well-being, recognizing that true health and wellness encompass all dimensions of human experience.

8. Sense of Transcendence and Wholeness:
- Spirituality offers a sense of transcendence and wholeness beyond the limitations of the ego and material existence. It invites individuals to explore the mysteries of existence, contemplate life's ultimate questions, and experience moments of awe, wonder, and reverence for the sacredness of life.

Practices for Cultivating Spiritual Wellness

Cultivating spiritual wellness involves engaging in practices that nurture your sense of meaning, purpose, connection, and inner peace. These practices can vary widely depending on individual beliefs, traditions, and preferences. Here are some practices for cultivating spiritual wellness:

1. Meditation and Mindfulness:

- Meditation and mindfulness practices involve cultivating present-moment awareness, inner calm, and clarity of mind. Regular meditation helps quiet the chatter of the mind, reduce stress, and deepen your connection to the present moment. Mindfulness practices can be integrated into daily activities such as walking, eating, and breathing, allowing you to cultivate awareness and presence in all aspects of life.

2. Prayer and Contemplation:

- Prayer, whether formal or informal, involves connecting with a higher power, divine source, or inner wisdom through communication, reflection, and surrender. Contemplative practices such as journaling, reflective writing, and silent reflection provide opportunities for introspection, self-inquiry, and spiritual exploration.

3. Connection with Nature:

- Spending time in nature can be a powerful way to cultivate spiritual wellness and connect with the natural world. Whether it's taking a walk in the woods, sitting by the ocean, or gardening in your backyard, immersing yourself in nature can evoke feelings of awe, gratitude, and reverence for the interconnectedness of all life.

4. Creative Expression:

- Engaging in creative activities such as art, music, dance, writing, and storytelling can be deeply nourishing for the soul. Creative expression allows you to tap into your inner wisdom, express your unique voice, and connect with the deeper aspects of your being.

5. Service and Compassion:

- Acts of service, kindness, and compassion toward others can be powerful ways to cultivate spiritual wellness and deepen your sense of connection and purpose. Volunteering, helping those in need, and practicing empathy and understanding foster a sense of interconnectedness and contribute to the well-being of both yourself and others.

6. Rituals and Ceremonies:

- Rituals and ceremonies provide structured opportunities for spiritual connection, meaning-making, and community. Whether it's lighting candles, offering prayers, celebrating holidays, or participating in sacred ceremonies, rituals can help you mark transitions, honor milestones, and cultivate a sense of sacredness in everyday life.

7. Study and Reflection:
   - Engaging in spiritual study, reading sacred texts, and exploring philosophical or religious teachings can deepen your understanding of spiritual principles and inspire personal growth and transformation. Reflecting on spiritual teachings, wisdom traditions, and life lessons can provide insights, guidance, and inspiration for your spiritual journey.

8. Gratitude and Mindful Living:
   - Cultivating an attitude of gratitude and practicing mindful living can foster spiritual wellness and enhance your appreciation for life's blessings. Taking time each day to count your blessings, express gratitude, and savor the present moment cultivates a sense of abundance, joy, and contentment.

9. Connection with Community:
   - Building supportive relationships and connecting with like-minded individuals can nourish your spiritual well-being and provide opportunities for shared growth, learning, and exploration. Participating in spiritual communities, gatherings, or support groups can provide encouragement, validation, and a sense of belonging on your spiritual journey.

10. Self-Care and Nurturing Practices:
   - Engaging in self-care practices that nourish your body, mind, and spirit is essential for spiritual wellness. Prioritize activities that replenish your energy, such as rest, relaxation, healthy eating, exercise, and time spent in activities that bring you joy and fulfillment.

Connecting with Nature and the Universe

Connecting with nature and the universe is a profound aspect of cultivating spiritual well-being. It involves recognizing the interconnectedness of all life, experiencing awe and wonder in the natural world, and fostering a sense of reverence and respect for the universe. Here are some practices for connecting with nature and the universe:

1. Spending Time Outdoors:
- Make time to immerse yourself in natural environments regularly. Whether it's a walk in the park, a hike in the mountains, or a stroll along the beach, spending time outdoors allows you to connect with the rhythms of nature, breathe fresh air, and rejuvenate your spirit.

2. Mindful Observation:
- Practice mindful observation of the natural world. Take time to notice the beauty and complexity of nature's patterns, colors, textures, and sounds. Observe the changing seasons, the movement of clouds, the growth of plants, and the behavior of animals with a sense of curiosity and wonder.

3. Nature Immersion:
- Engage in activities that allow you to fully immerse yourself in nature. Consider camping, backpacking, kayaking, birdwatching, or gardening as opportunities to deepen your connection with the natural world and experience a sense of awe and belonging.

4. Nature Meditation:
- Practice nature meditation by finding a quiet spot outdoors and sitting or walking mindfully. Use your senses to connect with your surroundings, focusing on the sights, sounds, smells, and sensations of nature. Allow yourself to be fully present and open to the beauty and wisdom of the natural world.

5. Earth-Based Rituals:
- Participate in earth-based rituals and ceremonies that honor the cycles of nature and the elements. Celebrate solstices, equinoxes, full moons, and other natural milestones with rituals such as ceremonies, prayers, offerings, and sacred practices that acknowledge the interconnectedness of all life.

6. Nature Journaling:

- Keep a nature journal to document your observations, reflections, and experiences in the natural world. Use writing, drawing, photography, or other creative means to capture moments of inspiration, insight, and connection with nature.

7. Environmental Stewardship:

- Engage in environmental stewardship and conservation efforts to protect and preserve the natural world. Get involved in community clean-up projects, tree planting initiatives, wildlife conservation programs, and advocacy campaigns that promote sustainability and ecological harmony.

8. Astrology and Astronomy:

- Explore the wonders of the universe through astrology and astronomy. Study the movements of celestial bodies, planetary alignments, and cosmic phenomena to deepen your understanding of the interconnectedness of the cosmos and the role of humanity within the vastness of space and time.

9. Star Gazing and Night Sky Observation:

- Spend time observing the night sky and connecting with the stars, planets, and galaxies above. Find a dark, quiet location away from city lights, and use telescopes, binoculars, or the naked eye to explore the mysteries of the cosmos and contemplate the infinite beauty and majesty of the universe.

10. Cultivating Gratitude and Reverence:

- Cultivate a sense of gratitude and reverence for the natural world and the universe. Practice expressing appreciation for the gifts of nature, the miracle of life, and the interconnected web of existence that sustains all living beings on Earth.

Holistic Approaches to Religion and Belief Systems

Holistic approaches to religion and belief systems recognize the importance of spirituality in promoting overall well-being while respecting the diversity of individual beliefs, practices, and cultural traditions. These approaches emphasize the integration of spiritual principles with physical, mental, and emotional health, fostering a sense of connection, meaning, and purpose in life. Here are some holistic approaches to religion and belief systems:

1. Respect for Diversity:
   - Embrace and celebrate the diversity of religious and spiritual beliefs, practices, and traditions. Recognize that there are many paths to spiritual growth and enlightenment, and honor the richness of human experience and cultural expression.

2. Integration of Mind, Body, and Spirit:
   - Recognize the interconnectedness of mind, body, and spirit in spiritual well-being. Emphasize practices that promote holistic health and integration, such as meditation, prayer, yoga, and mindfulness, which nurture spiritual awareness, physical vitality, and emotional resilience.

3. Promotion of Inner Peace and Harmony:
   - Encourage practices that cultivate inner peace, harmony, and balance. Teach mindfulness techniques, relaxation exercises, and stress reduction strategies that help individuals quiet the mind, soothe the spirit, and find tranquility amid life's challenges.

4. Empowerment and Self-Discovery:
   - Support individuals in their spiritual journey of self-discovery, growth, and transformation. Provide opportunities for introspection, self-reflection, and exploration of beliefs and values that resonate with personal truth and authenticity.

5. Community and Connection:
   - Foster a sense of community and connection among individuals with shared spiritual values and aspirations. Create opportunities for fellowship, support, and collaboration in spiritual practice, service, and social action that promote unity, compassion, and social justice.

6. Environmental Stewardship:
   - Promote environmental stewardship and reverence for the natural world as integral aspects of spiritual practice. Encourage sustainable living practices, ecological awareness, and respect for the

interconnectedness of all life, fostering a sense of responsibility and care for the Earth and future generations.

7. Service and Compassion:
- Emphasize the importance of service, altruism, and compassion as expressions of spiritual values and virtues. Engage in acts of kindness, generosity, and social responsibility that benefit others and contribute to the greater good, fostering a sense of purpose and fulfillment in life.

8. Integration of Science and Spirituality:
- Embrace an integrative approach that honors both scientific inquiry and spiritual wisdom. Recognize the complementarity of scientific knowledge and spiritual insight in understanding the mysteries of existence and the interconnectedness of all phenomena.

9. Cultivation of Gratitude and Reverence:
- Cultivate a sense of gratitude, reverence, and awe for the mysteries of life and the universe. Encourage practices that evoke wonder, appreciation, and humility in the face of the profound beauty, complexity, and interconnectedness of existence.

10. Promotion of Peace, Justice, and Well-Being:
- Advocate for peace, justice, and well-being as core values of spiritual practice and social transformation. Work towards creating a world that reflects the principles of compassion, equality, and dignity for all beings, fostering a culture of peace, harmony, and holistic well-being.

The Impact of Spiritual Health on Overall Well-Being

The impact of spiritual health on overall well-being is profound and multifaceted, encompassing physical, mental, emotional, and social aspects of health. Spiritual well-being contributes to a sense of meaning, purpose, connection, and inner peace, influencing various dimensions of an individual's overall well-being. Here are some key ways in which spiritual health impacts overall well-being:

1. **Enhanced Sense of Meaning and Purpose:**
   - Spiritual well-being provides individuals with a sense of meaning and purpose in life, helping them understand their place in the world and find significance in their experiences and relationships. Having a clear sense of purpose and direction contributes to overall life satisfaction and well-being.

2. **Improved Mental and Emotional Health:**
   - Spiritual practices such as meditation, prayer, and mindfulness have been shown to reduce stress, anxiety, and depression, promoting mental and emotional well-being. Cultivating spiritual resilience and coping skills helps individuals navigate life's challenges with greater ease and equanimity.

3. **Increased Resilience and Coping:**
   - Spiritual beliefs and practices foster resilience and coping abilities, helping individuals bounce back from adversity, trauma, and loss. Spiritual resources such as faith, hope, and optimism provide comfort, strength, and meaning during difficult times, supporting overall psychological resilience.

4. **Enhanced Quality of Relationships:**
   - Spiritual well-being fosters deeper connections and intimacy in relationships, promoting empathy, compassion, and forgiveness. Shared spiritual values and practices strengthen bonds with others, creating a sense of community, belonging, and support that enhances overall social well-being.

5. **Promotion of Physical Health:**
   - Spiritual practices such as meditation, prayer, and yoga have been linked to improvements in physical health outcomes such as lower blood pressure, reduced inflammation, and enhanced immune function. Spiritual well-being contributes to overall physical health by reducing stress-related illness and promoting holistic wellness.

6. **Greater Sense of Connection and Belonging:**
   - Spiritual well-being fosters a sense of connection and belonging to oneself, others, and the universe, promoting a feeling of

interconnectedness and unity. This sense of belonging enhances social support, reduces feelings of isolation, and contributes to overall emotional well-being.

7. Facilitation of Growth and Self-Actualization:

- Spiritual health facilitates personal growth, self-awareness, and self-actualization, helping individuals realize their full potential and live authentically. Spiritual practices encourage introspection, self-reflection, and exploration of values, beliefs, and aspirations that contribute to overall self-development and fulfillment.

8. Promotion of Compassion and Altruism:

- Spiritual well-being fosters qualities such as compassion, empathy, and altruism, promoting prosocial behavior and ethical conduct. Cultivating a compassionate heart and a sense of interconnectedness with all beings enhances social cohesion, cooperation, and collective well-being.

9. Reduction of Existential Distress:

- Spiritual well-being provides individuals with a framework for addressing existential questions and concerns about the meaning and purpose of life, death, and suffering. Spiritual beliefs and practices offer comfort, solace, and hope in the face of existential uncertainty, reducing existential distress and promoting inner peace.

10. Contribution to Overall Life Satisfaction and Fulfillment:

- Spiritual well-being contributes to overall life satisfaction and fulfillment by nurturing a sense of wholeness, harmony, and alignment with one's values, beliefs, and aspirations. Individuals with strong spiritual health report greater levels of subjective well-being, happiness, and overall life satisfaction.

Chapter 11
Holistic Perspectives on Illness and Disease

Viewing Illness Through a Holistic Lens

Viewing illness through a holistic lens involves recognizing that health and well-being are influenced by multiple interconnected factors, including physical, mental, emotional, social, environmental, and spiritual dimensions. Instead of focusing solely on symptoms and pathology, holistic perspectives on illness consider the whole person and the broader context in which illness arises. Here's how illness is viewed through a holistic lens:

1. **Mind-Body Connection:**
   - Holistic perspectives recognize the intimate connection between the mind and body, understanding that mental and emotional factors can profoundly impact physical health. Stress, negative emotions, trauma, and unresolved psychological issues can contribute to the onset and progression of illness. Addressing mental and emotional imbalances is essential for promoting holistic healing and restoring balance to the mind-body system.

2. **Root Causes vs. Symptoms:**
   - Holistic approaches prioritize identifying and addressing the underlying root causes of illness, rather than simply treating symptoms. Illness is viewed as a manifestation of imbalance or disharmony within the body-mind-spirit system, stemming from a combination of genetic, environmental, lifestyle, and psychosocial factors. Healing involves addressing these root causes and restoring balance to the whole person.

3. **Bio-Psycho-Social-Spiritual Model:**
   - Holistic perspectives on illness adopt a bio-psycho-social-spiritual model that considers the interplay of biological, psychological, social, and spiritual factors in health and disease. Illness is understood as a complex interaction between genetic predisposition, lifestyle factors, social determinants of health, and spiritual well-being. Healing requires addressing all aspects of the individual and their environment.

4. **Prevention and Wellness Promotion:**
   - Holistic approaches emphasize prevention and wellness promotion as essential components of health care. By addressing underlying

imbalances, promoting healthy lifestyle behaviors, and cultivating resilience and self-care practices, individuals can reduce their risk of illness and optimize their overall well-being.

5. Individualized and Person-Centered Care:
- Holistic care is individualized and person-centered, taking into account the unique needs, preferences, beliefs, and values of each individual. Treatment plans are tailored to address the whole person and may incorporate a variety of complementary and alternative therapies, conventional medical interventions, and lifestyle interventions to support healing and holistic wellness.

6. Empowerment and Self-Responsibility:
- Holistic perspectives empower individuals to take an active role in their health and healing process. By encouraging self-awareness, self-care practices, and self-empowerment, individuals can become active participants in their own healing journey and take responsibility for their health and well-being.

7. Integration of Complementary Therapies:
- Holistic approaches integrate complementary and alternative therapies alongside conventional medical treatments to address the physical, mental, emotional, and spiritual aspects of illness. Modalities such as acupuncture, herbal medicine, massage therapy, energy healing, mind-body practices, and spiritual counseling may be used to support holistic healing and enhance overall well-being.

8. Cultural Sensitivity and Diversity:
- Holistic perspectives on illness recognize the importance of cultural sensitivity and diversity in health care. Healing practices are respectful of cultural beliefs, traditions, and values, and honor the unique perspectives and experiences of individuals from diverse backgrounds. Culturally appropriate care promotes trust, collaboration, and mutual respect in the healing relationship.

9. Emphasis on Holistic Wellness:
- Holistic approaches to illness focus not only on treating disease but also on promoting holistic wellness and vitality. Healing involves fostering resilience, enhancing quality of life, and supporting

individuals in achieving their highest potential for health and well-being across the lifespan.

10. Interconnectedness and Interdependence:
   - Holistic perspectives recognize the interconnectedness and interdependence of all living beings and the environment. Illness is viewed within the broader context of ecological health, social justice, and planetary well-being, emphasizing the importance of sustainability, equity, and collective responsibility for creating conditions that support health and flourishing for all.

Mind-Body Approaches to Chronic Conditions

Mind-body approaches to chronic conditions are integral to holistic health, recognizing the interconnectedness of physical health, mental well-being, and emotional balance. These approaches focus on addressing not only the physical symptoms but also the underlying psychological, emotional, and lifestyle factors that contribute to chronic illness. Here are key mind-body approaches to managing chronic conditions:

1. Stress Reduction Techniques:
   - Chronic stress can exacerbate symptoms and contribute to the progression of chronic conditions. Mind-body techniques such as mindfulness meditation, deep breathing exercises, progressive muscle relaxation, and guided imagery help reduce stress levels, promote relaxation, and support overall well-being. Regular practice of these techniques can help individuals manage stress more effectively and alleviate symptoms associated with chronic illness.

2. Cognitive-Behavioral Therapy (CBT):
   - CBT is a psychotherapeutic approach that helps individuals identify and modify negative thought patterns, beliefs, and behaviors that contribute to chronic conditions. By addressing cognitive distortions, maladaptive coping strategies, and emotional triggers, CBT can help individuals manage pain, improve mood, and enhance quality of life. CBT techniques may include cognitive restructuring, relaxation training, and stress management strategies.

3. Mindfulness-Based Stress Reduction (MBSR):
- MBSR is a structured program that combines mindfulness meditation, yoga, and cognitive-behavioral techniques to reduce stress and improve coping with chronic illness and pain. Through mindfulness practices, participants learn to cultivate present-moment awareness, non-judgmental acceptance, and self-compassion, allowing them to navigate physical discomfort and emotional distress with greater ease and resilience.

4. Biofeedback and Relaxation Training:
- Biofeedback is a mind-body technique that helps individuals learn to control physiological processes such as heart rate, blood pressure, and muscle tension through self-regulation and feedback mechanisms. By monitoring and adjusting physiological responses, individuals can reduce symptoms related to chronic conditions such as hypertension, migraines, and chronic pain. Relaxation training techniques, including biofeedback-assisted relaxation, progressive muscle relaxation, and autogenic training, promote relaxation and stress reduction, enhancing overall well-being.

5. Yoga and Tai Chi:
- Yoga and Tai Chi are mind-body practices that combine physical postures, breathwork, and meditation to promote balance, flexibility, and relaxation. Both practices have been shown to improve symptoms and quality of life in individuals with chronic conditions such as arthritis, fibromyalgia, and chronic pain. Yoga and Tai Chi also enhance mental focus, emotional resilience, and spiritual well-being, supporting holistic health and wellness.

6. Art Therapy and Expressive Arts:
- Art therapy and expressive arts modalities provide creative outlets for individuals to explore and express their emotions, experiences, and innermost thoughts. Through painting, drawing, writing, music, dance, and other artistic mediums, individuals can process and integrate feelings related to their chronic condition, reduce anxiety and depression, and foster self-expression and empowerment.

7. Nutrition and Mindful Eating:

- Nutrition plays a crucial role in managing chronic conditions and promoting overall health and well-being. Mindful eating practices involve paying attention to hunger and satiety cues, savoring flavors and textures, and cultivating a non-judgmental awareness of food choices and eating behaviors. By practicing mindful eating, individuals can develop a healthier relationship with food, make more nourishing dietary choices, and manage symptoms related to chronic conditions such as diabetes, obesity, and gastrointestinal disorders.

8. Spiritual Support and Meaning-Making:

- Chronic illness often raises existential questions and challenges individuals' sense of meaning and purpose in life. Spiritual support and meaning-making practices, including prayer, meditation, and existential exploration, can provide comfort, solace, and a sense of transcendence amid the challenges of chronic illness. Spiritual practices help individuals find meaning, hope, and resilience in the face of adversity, supporting holistic healing and well-being.

9. Social Support and Community Engagement:

- Social support networks and community engagement play a vital role in managing chronic conditions and promoting holistic health. Connecting with others who share similar experiences, participating in support groups, and engaging in community activities provide emotional validation, practical assistance, and a sense of belonging that fosters resilience and well-being. Social support also buffers the negative effects of stress and enhances coping with chronic illness.

10. Holistic Lifestyle Interventions:

- Holistic lifestyle interventions encompass a range of mind-body practices, including exercise, sleep hygiene, stress management, and self-care strategies, that support overall health and well-being. By adopting a holistic approach to lifestyle, individuals can optimize physical health, enhance mental and emotional resilience, and reduce the impact of chronic conditions on their quality of life.

Integrative Medicine and Holistic Healthcare

Integrative medicine and holistic healthcare represent comprehensive approaches to healing that combine conventional medical treatments with complementary and alternative therapies, focusing on the whole person and addressing the underlying causes of illness. These approaches recognize the interconnectedness of body, mind, emotions, and spirit in promoting health and wellness. Here's an overview of integrative medicine and holistic healthcare:

1. Comprehensive Assessment and Individualized Treatment:
   - Integrative medicine and holistic healthcare practitioners conduct comprehensive assessments that consider physical, mental, emotional, social, environmental, and spiritual factors influencing health and well-being. Treatment plans are individualized and tailored to address the unique needs, preferences, and goals of each person, incorporating a range of evidence-based interventions and complementary therapies.

2. Collaborative and Multidisciplinary Care:
   - Integrative medicine and holistic healthcare emphasize collaboration and teamwork among healthcare providers from various disciplines, including physicians, nurses, therapists, nutritionists, acupuncturists, chiropractors, and mind-body practitioners. This multidisciplinary approach allows for the integration of diverse perspectives and expertise in addressing complex health issues and promoting holistic healing.

3. Focus on Prevention and Wellness Promotion:
   - Integrative medicine and holistic healthcare prioritize prevention and wellness promotion as essential components of healthcare. By identifying and addressing risk factors, promoting healthy lifestyle behaviors, and fostering resilience and self-care practices, these approaches aim to prevent illness, optimize health, and enhance overall well-being.

4. Use of Evidence-Based and Traditional Healing Modalities:
   - Integrative medicine and holistic healthcare integrate evidence-based conventional medical treatments with traditional healing modalities and complementary therapies. These may include acupuncture, herbal medicine, massage therapy, chiropractic care, mind-body practices, nutritional counseling, and energy healing

techniques, among others. By combining the best of both conventional and alternative approaches, integrative medicine offers a comprehensive toolkit for healing and wellness.

5. Emphasis on Patient-Centered Care and Empowerment:
- Integrative medicine and holistic healthcare prioritize patient-centered care and empowerment, emphasizing active participation, informed decision-making, and shared decision-making between patients and healthcare providers. Patients are encouraged to take an active role in their healing journey, make informed choices about their health, and become partners in their care, fostering a sense of ownership and empowerment.

6. Holistic Perspective on Illness and Healing:
- Integrative medicine and holistic healthcare view illness as a manifestation of imbalance or disharmony within the body-mind-spirit system, stemming from a combination of genetic, environmental, lifestyle, and psychosocial factors. Healing involves addressing the underlying root causes of illness, restoring balance to the whole person, and supporting the body's innate capacity for self-healing and self-regulation.

7. Promotion of Self-Care and Self-Healing:
- Integrative medicine and holistic healthcare promote self-care and self-healing practices that empower individuals to take an active role in maintaining their health and well-being. These may include stress management techniques, mindfulness practices, healthy eating habits, regular exercise, adequate sleep, and mind-body interventions that support holistic wellness and resilience.

8. Emotional and Psychological Support:
- Integrative medicine and holistic healthcare recognize the importance of addressing emotional and psychological factors in health and healing. Therapeutic approaches such as counseling, psychotherapy, mindfulness-based interventions, and expressive arts therapies help individuals process emotions, cope with stress, and cultivate resilience, contributing to overall well-being and quality of life.

9. Promotion of Environmental and Planetary Health:

   - Integrative medicine and holistic healthcare acknowledge the interconnectedness of human health with environmental and planetary health. These approaches advocate for sustainable living practices, environmental stewardship, and social responsibility to create conditions that support health and well-being for individuals, communities, and the planet as a whole.

10. Research and Education:

   - Integrative medicine and holistic healthcare support ongoing research and education to advance understanding of holistic approaches to health and healing. By conducting rigorous scientific studies, disseminating evidence-based information, and training healthcare professionals in integrative and holistic practices, these approaches contribute to the evolution of healthcare towards a more holistic, patient-centered, and sustainable model of care.

Holistic Cancer Care

Holistic cancer care encompasses a comprehensive approach to addressing the physical, emotional, mental, social, and spiritual aspects of cancer diagnosis, treatment, and survivorship. It integrates conventional medical treatments with complementary and alternative therapies to support the whole person throughout the cancer journey. Here's an overview of holistic cancer care:

1. Comprehensive Assessment and Individualized Treatment:

   - Holistic cancer care begins with a thorough assessment of the individual's medical history, cancer diagnosis, treatment options, and overall health status. Treatment plans are tailored to the unique needs, preferences, and goals of each patient, incorporating a combination of conventional cancer treatments, complementary therapies, and supportive care interventions.

2. Collaborative and Multidisciplinary Approach:

   - Holistic cancer care involves collaboration among a multidisciplinary team of healthcare providers, including oncologists, surgeons, nurses, nutritionists, psychologists, social workers, and complementary therapists. This team-based approach ensures coordinated care, holistic support, and personalized treatment strategies that address the physical, emotional, and psychosocial needs of cancer patients.

3. Integration of Conventional and Complementary Therapies:
   - Holistic cancer care integrates evidence-based conventional cancer treatments such as surgery, chemotherapy, radiation therapy, and targeted therapy with complementary and alternative therapies such as acupuncture, massage therapy, yoga, meditation, nutritional counseling, and mind-body interventions. These complementary therapies can help manage treatment side effects, alleviate symptoms, improve quality of life, and support overall well-being during and after cancer treatment.

4. Focus on Symptom Management and Quality of Life:
   - Holistic cancer care prioritizes symptom management, supportive care, and quality of life throughout the cancer journey. Therapies such as acupuncture, massage, and integrative pain management techniques can help alleviate pain, fatigue, nausea, and other treatment-related side effects, improving overall well-being and treatment tolerance. Emotional support, counseling, and psychotherapy are also offered to help patients cope with the psychological and emotional impact of cancer diagnosis and treatment.

5. Nutritional Support and Lifestyle Interventions:
   - Holistic cancer care emphasizes the importance of nutrition, exercise, and lifestyle interventions in supporting overall health and well-being during and after cancer treatment. Nutritionists and dietitians provide guidance on healthy eating habits, dietary supplements, and nutritional strategies to optimize immune function, support healing, and reduce the risk of cancer recurrence. Exercise programs tailored to individual needs and preferences help improve physical fitness, reduce fatigue, and enhance quality of life for cancer survivors.

6. Emotional and Psychosocial Support:
   - Holistic cancer care recognizes the emotional and psychosocial impact of cancer diagnosis and treatment on patients and their

families. Psychologists, social workers, and counselors offer emotional support, coping skills training, and supportive therapy to help patients navigate the emotional challenges, fears, and uncertainties associated with cancer. Support groups, peer counseling, and survivorship programs provide opportunities for connection, camaraderie, and shared experiences among cancer survivors.

7. Mind-Body Interventions and Stress Reduction Techniques:
   - Holistic cancer care incorporates mind-body interventions and stress reduction techniques to promote relaxation, emotional balance, and resilience during the cancer journey. Mindfulness-based stress reduction (MBSR), guided imagery, relaxation exercises, and expressive arts therapies help patients reduce stress, manage anxiety, and enhance coping skills, fostering a sense of inner peace and well-being amidst the challenges of cancer treatment.

8. Spiritual and Existential Support:
   - Holistic cancer care addresses the spiritual and existential dimensions of the cancer experience, providing opportunities for reflection, meaning-making, and spiritual support. Chaplains, pastoral counselors, and spiritual care providers offer spiritual guidance, rituals, and support to help patients find hope, meaning, and transcendence in the face of cancer diagnosis, treatment, and survivorship.

9. Survivorship and Rehabilitation Programs:
   - Holistic cancer care includes survivorship and rehabilitation programs designed to support patients during the transition from active treatment to survivorship. These programs address the long-term physical, emotional, and psychosocial needs of cancer survivors, providing resources, education, and support to help them thrive beyond cancer.

10. Empowerment and Advocacy:
   - Holistic cancer care empowers patients to take an active role in their treatment decisions, self-care practices, and survivorship journey. Patient education, advocacy resources, and empowerment programs help patients become informed, empowered advocates for their own health and well-being, fostering a sense of agency, autonomy, and resilience in the face of cancer.

Holistic Perspectives on Mental Health Disorders

Holistic perspectives on mental health disorders recognize the interconnectedness of biological, psychological, social, environmental, and spiritual factors in the development, manifestation, and treatment of mental illness. These perspectives emphasize a comprehensive approach to mental health care that addresses the whole person and considers multiple dimensions of health and well-being. Here are key components of holistic perspectives on mental health disorders:

1. **Biopsychosocial-Spiritual Model:**
   - Holistic perspectives on mental health disorders adopt a biopsychosocial-spiritual model that acknowledges the complex interplay of biological, psychological, social, and spiritual factors in mental illness. Rather than focusing solely on biological or psychological factors, these perspectives consider the influence of social determinants, environmental stressors, and spiritual beliefs on mental health and well-being.

2. **Mind-Body Connection:**
   - Holistic approaches to mental health recognize the intimate connection between the mind and body, understanding that mental and emotional well-being are influenced by physical health and vice versa. Imbalances in neurotransmitters, hormones, and physiological processes can contribute to the development of mental health disorders, while psychological factors such as stress, trauma, and negative thought patterns can affect physical health and exacerbate symptoms of mental illness.

3. **Root Causes vs. Symptoms:**
   - Holistic perspectives prioritize identifying and addressing the underlying root causes of mental health disorders, rather than simply treating symptoms. These root causes may include genetic predisposition, biochemical imbalances, unresolved trauma, adverse childhood experiences, dysfunctional relationships, environmental toxins, and spiritual disconnection. Healing involves addressing these underlying factors and restoring balance to the whole person.

4. Emphasis on Prevention and Wellness Promotion:
   - Holistic approaches to mental health emphasize prevention and wellness promotion as essential components of mental health care. Strategies for prevention may include early intervention, education, screening, and addressing risk factors such as stress, trauma, substance abuse, and social isolation. Wellness promotion focuses on cultivating resilience, coping skills, self-care practices, and healthy lifestyle behaviors that support mental well-being.

5. Integration of Conventional and Complementary Therapies:
   - Holistic perspectives on mental health embrace a wide range of treatment modalities, including both conventional psychiatric treatments and complementary and alternative therapies. Conventional treatments such as medication, psychotherapy, and hospitalization may be integrated with complementary approaches such as mindfulness-based interventions, acupuncture, yoga, nutrition counseling, art therapy, and energy healing techniques.

6. Individualized and Person-Centered Care:
   - Holistic mental health care is individualized and person-centered, taking into account the unique needs, preferences, strengths, and values of each individual. Treatment plans are tailored to address the specific symptoms, challenges, and goals of the person, with a focus on fostering autonomy, empowerment, and collaboration in the healing process.

7. Holistic Lifestyle Interventions:
   - Holistic approaches to mental health emphasize the importance of lifestyle interventions in promoting mental well-being. These may include strategies for improving sleep hygiene, nutrition, exercise, stress management, social support, and spiritual connection. Lifestyle interventions support overall health and resilience, reduce the risk of mental health disorders, and enhance the effectiveness of other treatment modalities.

8. Social and Environmental Factors:
   - Holistic perspectives on mental health consider the impact of social and environmental factors on mental well-being. Socioeconomic status,

cultural norms, family dynamics, community support, housing stability, access to healthcare, and environmental stressors such as pollution and urbanization can all influence mental health outcomes. Addressing social and environmental determinants of health is essential for promoting equity, social justice, and mental health for all.

9. Spiritual and Existential Support:
 - Holistic mental health care recognizes the importance of addressing spiritual and existential dimensions of mental illness. Chaplains, pastoral counselors, and spiritual care providers offer support and guidance to individuals grappling with questions of meaning, purpose, identity, and faith in the context of mental health challenges. Spiritual practices such as meditation, prayer, and contemplation can provide comfort, solace, and a sense of transcendence amid the struggles of mental illness.

10. Community and Peer Support:
 - Holistic mental health care values the role of community and peer support in promoting recovery, resilience, and social connection. Support groups, peer-led initiatives, mutual aid networks, and community-based organizations provide opportunities for validation, empathy, understanding, and shared experiences among individuals with mental health disorders. Peer support fosters a sense of belonging, acceptance, and hope that is essential for healing and recovery.

Chapter 12
Holistic Approaches to Women's Health

Holistic Perspectives on Women's Wellness

Holistic approaches to women's health encompass a comprehensive view of well-being that addresses the physical, emotional, mental, social, and spiritual aspects unique to women. These perspectives recognize the interconnectedness of various factors in influencing women's health and wellness throughout their lives. Here's an overview of holistic perspectives on women's wellness:

1. **Hormonal Balance and Reproductive Health:**
   - Holistic approaches to women's health emphasize the importance of hormonal balance and reproductive health in supporting overall well-being. These perspectives recognize the influence of hormonal fluctuations throughout the menstrual cycle, pregnancy, childbirth, and menopause on women's physical health, emotional stability, and mental well-being. Holistic interventions may include nutritional support, lifestyle modifications, herbal remedies, and mind-body practices to promote hormonal balance and reproductive vitality.

2. **Preventive Care and Wellness Promotion:**
   - Holistic perspectives prioritize preventive care and wellness promotion as essential components of women's health. Strategies for prevention may include regular health screenings, immunizations, health education, and lifestyle interventions that support healthy aging, disease prevention, and early detection of health issues. Holistic wellness programs offer resources, education, and support to help women maintain optimal health and well-being throughout their lives.

3. **Menstrual Health and Menstrual Cycle Awareness:**
   - Holistic approaches to women's health honor the menstrual cycle as a natural, cyclical process that reflects women's hormonal, emotional, and energetic rhythms. Menstrual health practices involve menstrual cycle tracking, menstrual hygiene management, and menstrual cycle awareness to promote self-awareness, self-care, and empowerment around women's reproductive health. These practices help women better understand their bodies, identify patterns, and make informed choices about their health and well-being.

4. **Pregnancy, Birth, and Postpartum Support:**

- Holistic perspectives on women's health recognize pregnancy, childbirth, and postpartum as transformative experiences that impact women physically, emotionally, mentally, and spiritually. Holistic maternity care emphasizes personalized, woman-centered care that honors women's autonomy, preferences, and cultural beliefs. Supportive care during pregnancy, birth, and postpartum may include nutritional counseling, childbirth education, labor support, breastfeeding support, and postpartum mental health care to promote a positive pregnancy and childbirth experience.

5. Nutrition and Lifestyle Interventions:

- Holistic approaches to women's health emphasize the importance of nutrition, exercise, and lifestyle interventions in supporting women's overall health and wellness. Nutritional strategies may include whole foods-based diets, supplementation, mindful eating practices, and herbal remedies to address specific women's health concerns such as menstrual irregularities, fertility issues, hormonal imbalances, and menopausal symptoms. Lifestyle interventions such as regular physical activity, stress management, adequate sleep, and social support also play a key role in promoting women's well-being.

6. Emotional and Psychological Well-Being:

- Holistic perspectives on women's health acknowledge the influence of emotional and psychological factors on women's health and wellness. Mental health care for women may involve counseling, therapy, support groups, and mind-body interventions to address issues such as anxiety, depression, trauma, grief, and relationship challenges. Holistic approaches emphasize self-care practices, self-awareness, and self-compassion to support women's emotional resilience, empowerment, and inner healing.

7. Social Determinants of Health and Equity:

- Holistic approaches to women's health recognize the impact of social determinants of health, including socioeconomic status, education, race, ethnicity, gender identity, sexual orientation, and access to healthcare, on women's health outcomes. These perspectives advocate for health equity, social justice, and culturally competent care that addresses systemic barriers and promotes inclusive, accessible, and equitable healthcare for all women.

8. Integrative and Complementary Therapies:

   - Holistic approaches to women's health integrate conventional medical treatments with complementary and alternative therapies to support women's health and wellness. Complementary therapies such as acupuncture, massage therapy, herbal medicine, chiropractic care, and mind-body practices offer additional options for managing women's health concerns and enhancing overall well-being. Integrative healthcare models provide collaborative, multidisciplinary care that addresses the whole person and integrates evidence-based interventions from diverse healing traditions.

9. Spiritual and Relational Wellness:

   - Holistic perspectives on women's health acknowledge the importance of spiritual and relational wellness in promoting holistic well-being. Spiritual practices such as meditation, prayer, ritual, and connection with nature offer opportunities for women to cultivate inner peace, resilience, and spiritual connection. Healthy relationships, community support, and social connections also play a vital role in women's emotional fulfillment, social support, and overall quality of life.

10. Empowerment and Advocacy:

   - Holistic approaches to women's health empower women to take an active role in their health and wellness journey, advocating for their own needs, preferences, and rights. Women's health education, empowerment programs, and advocacy initiatives promote informed decision-making, self-advocacy, and collective action to address women's health disparities, promote health equity, and advance women's rights and reproductive justice.

Natural Approaches to Reproductive Health

Natural approaches to reproductive health encompass a range of holistic strategies aimed at promoting fertility, supporting reproductive function, and enhancing overall well-being in women. These approaches emphasize lifestyle modifications, nutritional support, herbal remedies, mind-body practices, and environmental considerations to optimize reproductive health naturally. Here are key components of natural approaches to reproductive health for women:

1. Nutrition and Dietary Support:
   - A nutritious diet rich in essential vitamins, minerals, antioxidants, and phytonutrients is fundamental for reproductive health. Women should focus on consuming whole foods, including fruits, vegetables, whole grains, lean proteins, and healthy fats, while minimizing processed foods, sugar, caffeine, and alcohol. Specific nutrients such as folate, iron, omega-3 fatty acids, and antioxidants are particularly important for supporting fertility, hormonal balance, and reproductive function.

2. Hormonal Balance:
   - Hormonal imbalances can affect menstrual cycles, ovulation, and fertility. Natural approaches to hormonal balance may involve dietary modifications, stress management techniques, regular exercise, adequate sleep, and targeted nutritional supplementation. Certain herbs such as chasteberry (Vitex agnus-castus), maca root (Lepidium meyenii), and evening primrose oil (Oenothera biennis) are commonly used to support hormonal balance and regulate menstrual cycles.

3. Stress Reduction and Mind-Body Practices:
   - Chronic stress can disrupt hormonal balance and impair reproductive function. Mind-body practices such as yoga, meditation, deep breathing exercises, progressive muscle relaxation, and mindfulness-based stress reduction (MBSR) can help reduce stress levels, promote relaxation, and support emotional well-being. These practices can also enhance fertility by reducing the negative impact of stress on reproductive hormones and menstrual cycles.

4. Herbal Medicine and Phytotherapy:
   - Herbal medicine offers a rich tradition of botanical remedies that support reproductive health and fertility. Herbs such as red clover (Trifolium pratense), raspberry leaf (Rubus idaeus), dong quai (Angelica sinensis), and black cohosh (Actaea racemosa) are commonly used to regulate menstrual cycles, promote ovulation, and support overall reproductive function. Herbal formulations may be tailored to address

specific concerns such as hormonal imbalances, menstrual irregularities, and fertility challenges.

5. Acupuncture and Traditional Chinese Medicine (TCM):

   - Acupuncture and TCM offer holistic approaches to reproductive health that focus on restoring balance and harmony within the body. Acupuncture treatments target specific acupoints related to reproductive organs and hormonal regulation, aiming to improve blood flow, support ovarian function, and enhance fertility. Traditional Chinese herbal formulas may also be prescribed to address underlying imbalances and optimize reproductive health.

6. Environmental Toxin Reduction:

   - Exposure to environmental toxins such as endocrine-disrupting chemicals (EDCs) can negatively impact reproductive health and fertility. Natural approaches to reproductive health include minimizing exposure to environmental toxins found in plastics, personal care products, household cleaners, and pesticides. Choosing organic foods, using non-toxic household products, and filtering drinking water can help reduce exposure to harmful chemicals and support reproductive wellness.

7. Regular Physical Activity:

   - Regular exercise is beneficial for overall health and may positively impact reproductive function and fertility. Moderate-intensity exercise, such as brisk walking, swimming, cycling, or yoga, can help maintain a healthy weight, improve circulation, reduce stress, and support hormonal balance. However, excessive or intense exercise may disrupt menstrual cycles and ovulation, so it's important to find a balance that supports reproductive health.

8. Optimizing Sleep Quality:

   - Adequate sleep is essential for hormonal balance, immune function, and overall well-being. Natural approaches to reproductive health include optimizing sleep hygiene practices to ensure restorative sleep. This may involve establishing a regular sleep schedule, creating a relaxing bedtime routine, minimizing exposure to screens before bedtime, and creating a comfortable sleep environment conducive to quality rest.

9. Holistic Fertility Awareness Methods:
   - Holistic fertility awareness methods, such as tracking basal body temperature, cervical mucus changes, and menstrual cycle patterns, can help women gain insight into their fertility and menstrual cycles. By becoming more aware of their natural fertility signs, women can identify fertile windows for conception, monitor reproductive health, and make informed decisions about family planning and reproductive care.

10. Collaborative Care and Individualized Support:
   - Natural approaches to reproductive health often involve collaborative care and individualized support from healthcare providers who specialize in holistic and integrative medicine. Naturopathic doctors, functional medicine practitioners, herbalists, acupuncturists, and fertility specialists may work together to provide comprehensive care that addresses the unique needs and goals of each woman. By integrating conventional and complementary therapies, these providers offer personalized treatment plans that support women's reproductive health and fertility naturally.

Holistic Pregnancy and Childbirth

Holistic pregnancy and childbirth encompass a comprehensive approach to supporting women's physical, emotional, mental, and spiritual well-being throughout the prenatal, birthing, and postpartum periods. These approaches prioritize personalized care, informed decision-making, empowerment, and the integration of conventional and complementary therapies to optimize maternal and infant health outcomes. Here's an overview of holistic perspectives on pregnancy and childbirth:

1. Preconception Care and Fertility Optimization:
   - Holistic pregnancy begins with preconception care and fertility optimization, focusing on preparing the body for a healthy pregnancy. This may involve nutritional counseling, lifestyle modifications, stress reduction techniques, and environmental toxin avoidance to support hormonal balance, reproductive function, and overall well-being. Holistic practitioners offer personalized recommendations to address

underlying health issues, optimize fertility, and enhance the likelihood of conception.

2. Prenatal Nutrition and Wellness:
   - Proper nutrition and wellness during pregnancy are essential for maternal health and fetal development. Holistic approaches emphasize whole foods-based diets rich in essential nutrients such as folate, iron, calcium, omega-3 fatty acids, and antioxidants. Prenatal supplements, herbal remedies, and traditional foods may be recommended to meet increased nutritional needs and support optimal maternal-fetal health. Mindful eating practices, hydration, regular physical activity, and adequate rest are also important components of holistic prenatal care.

3. Emotional and Psychological Support:
   - Holistic pregnancy care addresses the emotional and psychological aspects of pregnancy, offering support and resources to help women navigate the emotional ups and downs of pregnancy. Counseling, therapy, support groups, and mind-body practices such as meditation, relaxation techniques, and visualization exercises can help women manage stress, anxiety, fears, and mood fluctuations during pregnancy. Holistic practitioners provide compassionate care, validation, and empowerment to women as they prepare for childbirth and parenthood.

4. Comprehensive Prenatal Care:
   - Holistic prenatal care involves regular check-ups, screenings, and assessments to monitor maternal and fetal health throughout pregnancy. In addition to standard medical care, holistic practitioners may offer complementary therapies such as acupuncture, chiropractic care, massage therapy, and naturopathic treatments to address common pregnancy-related discomforts, promote relaxation, and support overall well-being. Collaborative care between obstetricians, midwives, doulas, and other healthcare providers ensures a holistic and integrated approach to prenatal care.

5. Empowered Birth Planning:
   - Holistic approaches to childbirth empower women to make informed decisions about their birth preferences, goals, and desires. Birth planning involves exploring various options for labor and delivery,

discussing pain management strategies, and creating a birth plan that reflects the woman's values, wishes, and preferences. Holistic childbirth education classes, birth preparation workshops, and doula support provide valuable information, resources, and emotional support to women and their partners as they prepare for childbirth.

6. Natural and Mindful Birth Practices:

   - Holistic childbirth embraces natural and mindful birth practices that prioritize the physiological process of labor and birth. Techniques such as breathing exercises, relaxation techniques, movement, positioning, hydrotherapy, and massage can help women cope with labor pain, promote comfort, and facilitate the progress of labor. Holistic birth environments, including birth centers and home births, offer women the freedom to move, eat, drink, and labor in a supportive and empowering atmosphere.

7. Supportive Birth Environment:

   - Holistic childbirth emphasizes the importance of creating a supportive birth environment that respects the woman's autonomy, preferences, and choices. Continuous emotional support from a birth partner, doula, or support person can enhance women's sense of safety, security, and empowerment during labor and birth. Holistic birth settings prioritize privacy, autonomy, and dignity, providing a calm, peaceful, and nurturing atmosphere conducive to a positive birth experience.

8. Postpartum Recovery and Wellness:

   - Holistic postpartum care focuses on supporting women's physical and emotional recovery after childbirth, promoting bonding with the baby, and facilitating the transition to parenthood. Holistic practitioners offer postpartum check-ups, lactation support, nutritional counseling, emotional support, and resources for managing postpartum challenges such as sleep deprivation, breastfeeding issues, mood fluctuations, and physical recovery. Holistic postpartum care acknowledges the unique needs of each woman and provides compassionate, individualized support to promote postpartum healing and well-being.

9. Breastfeeding Support and Education:

- Holistic approaches to breastfeeding emphasize the importance of breastfeeding as a natural and beneficial way to nourish and bond with the baby. Breastfeeding support groups, lactation consultants, and peer counseling provide education, encouragement, and practical assistance to women who choose to breastfeed. Holistic lactation care addresses common breastfeeding challenges, promotes successful breastfeeding outcomes, and fosters a supportive breastfeeding relationship between mother and baby.

10. **Integration of Conventional and Complementary Therapies:**
   - Holistic pregnancy and childbirth integrate conventional medical care with complementary therapies to support women's health and well-being. While medical interventions may be necessary in certain circumstances, holistic approaches offer additional options for pain management, relaxation, comfort, and support throughout the childbirth process. Collaboration between obstetricians, midwives, doulas, and other healthcare providers ensures a comprehensive, woman-centered approach to pregnancy and childbirth that honors women's choices, preferences, and autonomy.

Nurturing Holistic Health Throughout the Menstrual Cycle

Nurturing holistic health throughout the menstrual cycle involves recognizing and honoring the natural rhythms and changes that occur in a woman's body and mind throughout each phase of her cycle. By adopting holistic approaches to women's health that align with the menstrual cycle, women can optimize their well-being, support hormonal balance, and enhance overall health and vitality. Here's how to nurture holistic health throughout the menstrual cycle:

1. Menstruation (Days 1-5):
   - During menstruation, women can prioritize rest, relaxation, and self-care practices to honor their body's need for rejuvenation and renewal. This may involve getting adequate rest, practicing gentle movement such as walking or yoga, staying hydrated, and nourishing the body with nutrient-rich foods. Women can also use this time for

introspection, journaling, and connecting with their inner wisdom and intuition.

2. Follicular Phase (Days 1-14):
 - The follicular phase is a time of renewal and growth, characterized by rising estrogen levels and the maturation of ovarian follicles. Women can support holistic health during this phase by focusing on activities that promote vitality, creativity, and new beginnings. This may include engaging in regular exercise, exploring new hobbies or interests, nourishing the body with fresh fruits and vegetables, and spending time in nature to connect with the energy of renewal and growth.

3. Ovulation (Approximately Day 14):
 - Ovulation marks the peak of fertility and vitality in the menstrual cycle, driven by a surge in luteinizing hormone (LH) and estrogen. Women can nurture holistic health during ovulation by embracing their sensuality, creativity, and connection to life. This may involve engaging in intimate relationships, expressing creativity through art or dance, and savoring pleasurable experiences. Supporting hormonal balance with nutrient-dense foods, adequate hydration, and stress reduction techniques can also enhance overall well-being during this phase.

4. Luteal Phase (Days 15-28):
 - The luteal phase is a time of preparation for potential pregnancy, characterized by increased progesterone levels and metabolic activity. Women can support holistic health during this phase by prioritizing self-care practices that promote relaxation, balance, and nourishment. This may include practicing stress reduction techniques such as meditation or deep breathing, incorporating gentle exercise such as yoga or Pilates, and focusing on nutrient-dense foods that support hormonal balance and stable blood sugar levels.

5. Premenstrual Phase (Days 25-28):
 - The premenstrual phase, also known as the luteal phase transition, is a time of introspection, reflection, and emotional processing as the body prepares for menstruation. Women can nurture holistic health during this phase by practicing self-compassion, self-care, and emotional resilience. This may involve engaging in activities that

promote relaxation and stress relief, such as spending time in nature, practicing mindfulness or meditation, and connecting with supportive friends or loved ones.

6. Cycle Awareness and Mind-Body Connection:
   - Throughout the menstrual cycle, women can cultivate cycle awareness and a deeper connection to their body's natural rhythms and signals. Holistic health practices such as cycle tracking, journaling, and mindfulness meditation can help women tune into their menstrual cycle's unique patterns and fluctuations, empowering them to make informed choices about their health and well-being. By honoring the body's innate wisdom and respecting its natural cycles, women can nurture holistic health throughout the menstrual cycle and beyond.

7. Nutrition and Lifestyle Support:
   - Supporting holistic health throughout the menstrual cycle involves adopting nutrition and lifestyle practices that promote hormonal balance, vitality, and well-being. Women can nourish their bodies with whole, nutrient-dense foods, staying hydrated, and minimizing processed foods, sugar, and caffeine. Regular physical activity, adequate sleep, stress management techniques, and social support also play essential roles in supporting holistic health throughout the menstrual cycle.

8. Emotional and Spiritual Wellness:
   - Holistic health encompasses emotional and spiritual well-being, which are integral aspects of women's health throughout the menstrual cycle. Women can nurture emotional wellness by practicing self-care, setting boundaries, and seeking support when needed. Spiritual practices such as meditation, prayer, or connecting with nature can provide a sense of grounding, purpose, and connection to something greater than oneself, supporting holistic health on a deeper level.

Integrating Mind-Body-Spirit Practices for Women's Well-Being

Integrating mind-body-spirit practices is essential for promoting holistic health and well-being in women. These practices recognize the interconnectedness of the mind, body, and spirit, and aim to foster balance, harmony, and vitality in all aspects of a woman's life. By incorporating mind-body-spirit practices into daily life, women can cultivate self-awareness, resilience, and inner peace, leading to greater overall well-being. Here are some key practices for integrating mind-body-spirit approaches for women's health:

1. Meditation and Mindfulness:
   - Meditation and mindfulness practices cultivate present-moment awareness, calm the mind, and reduce stress levels. Women can integrate meditation into their daily routine by setting aside time for quiet reflection, deep breathing exercises, or guided meditation sessions. Mindfulness techniques such as body scans, mindful walking, and mindful eating can help women connect with their bodies and surroundings, fostering a sense of inner peace and clarity.

2. Yoga and Tai Chi:
   - Yoga and Tai Chi are mind-body practices that combine movement, breathwork, and mindfulness to promote physical, mental, and emotional well-being. Women can benefit from regular yoga or Tai Chi practice to increase flexibility, strength, and balance, while also reducing stress, anxiety, and tension. These practices offer a holistic approach to fitness and wellness, supporting women's overall health and vitality.

3. Breathwork and Relaxation Techniques:
   - Breathwork and relaxation techniques help women manage stress, anxiety, and emotional overwhelm by activating the body's relaxation response. Deep breathing exercises, progressive muscle relaxation, and guided imagery can promote relaxation, reduce muscle tension, and calm the nervous system. Women can incorporate these practices into their daily routine or use them as tools to cope with challenging situations and promote emotional well-being.

4. Journaling and Creative Expression:
   - Journaling and creative expression provide outlets for self-reflection, self-expression, and emotional processing. Women can use journaling prompts, free writing, or art therapy techniques to explore their thoughts, feelings, and experiences, gaining insight into their

inner world and fostering self-awareness. Creative activities such as painting, drawing, or crafting can also serve as meditative practices, promoting relaxation and stress relief.

5. Nature Connection and Grounding Practices:

- Spending time in nature and connecting with the natural world can be deeply grounding and nourishing for women's well-being. Women can cultivate a connection to nature by spending time outdoors, practicing forest bathing, gardening, or engaging in outdoor activities such as hiking or camping. Grounding practices such as barefoot walking, earthing, or tree meditation can also help women feel more centered, balanced, and connected to the earth.

6. Spiritual Exploration and Connection:

- Spiritual practices such as prayer, meditation, ritual, or connecting with one's higher self or divine source can nourish the soul and provide a sense of meaning, purpose, and connection. Women can explore their spirituality through various practices that resonate with their beliefs and values, whether through organized religion, personal rituals, or spiritual communities. Cultivating a sense of spiritual connection can support women's mental and emotional well-being, providing comfort and guidance in challenging times.

7. Community and Support Networks:

- Building supportive relationships and community connections is vital for women's holistic health and well-being. Women can seek out supportive networks, women's circles, or community groups where they can connect with like-minded individuals, share experiences, and receive support and encouragement. Social connections provide emotional support, validation, and a sense of belonging, which are essential for overall well-being.

8. Self-Care and Self-Compassion:

- Practicing self-care and self-compassion is essential for women's well-being, as it allows them to prioritize their needs, set boundaries, and nurture themselves on all levels. Women can cultivate self-compassion through practices such as self-kindness, mindfulness, and self-acceptance, treating themselves with the same kindness and understanding they would offer to a friend. By making self-care a priority and honoring their own needs, women can replenish their energy, reduce burnout, and enhance their overall well-being.

Chapter 13
Holistic Perspectives on Men's Health

Holistic Approaches to Men's Wellness

Holistic approaches to men's wellness encompass a comprehensive and integrative approach to health that addresses the physical, mental, emotional, and spiritual aspects of well-being. These approaches recognize the interconnectedness of various factors in men's lives and aim to promote balance, vitality, and longevity. Here are key holistic approaches to men's wellness:

1. **Nutrition and Dietary Support:**
   - Holistic approaches to men's wellness emphasize the importance of a balanced and nutrient-rich diet to support overall health. Men are encouraged to consume whole foods such as fruits, vegetables, lean proteins, whole grains, and healthy fats, while minimizing processed foods, sugar, and unhealthy fats. Specific nutrients such as vitamins, minerals, antioxidants, and phytonutrients play essential roles in supporting men's health, hormone balance, and vitality.

2. **Physical Activity and Exercise:**
   - Regular physical activity and exercise are crucial components of men's wellness, promoting cardiovascular health, muscle strength, flexibility, and overall fitness. Holistic approaches encourage a variety of activities, including aerobic exercise, strength training, flexibility exercises, and mind-body practices such as yoga or Tai Chi. Men are encouraged to find activities they enjoy and incorporate them into their daily routine to support physical health and well-being.

3. **Stress Management and Mindfulness:**
   - Holistic approaches to men's wellness emphasize the importance of stress management techniques and mindfulness practices to support mental and emotional well-being. Men are encouraged to practice relaxation techniques such as deep breathing, meditation, progressive muscle relaxation, or guided imagery to reduce stress levels, promote relaxation, and improve overall mood. Mindfulness practices help men cultivate present-moment awareness, resilience, and emotional balance in the face of life's challenges.

4. **Sleep Hygiene and Restorative Sleep:**

- Quality sleep is essential for men's overall health and well-being, supporting physical, mental, and emotional functions. Holistic approaches to men's wellness emphasize the importance of sleep hygiene practices to promote restorative sleep. Men are encouraged to establish a regular sleep schedule, create a relaxing bedtime routine, optimize their sleep environment, and prioritize adequate sleep duration to support optimal health and vitality.

5. Social Connections and Support Networks:

- Building supportive relationships and social connections is essential for men's wellness, providing emotional support, companionship, and a sense of belonging. Holistic approaches encourage men to cultivate meaningful relationships with family, friends, and community members, and to seek out support networks or men's groups where they can connect with others who share similar interests and experiences.

6. Emotional Intelligence and Self-Awareness:

- Holistic approaches to men's wellness promote emotional intelligence and self-awareness as essential components of overall health and well-being. Men are encouraged to cultivate skills such as self-reflection, empathy, communication, and emotional regulation to enhance their relationships, cope with stress, and navigate life's challenges more effectively. Developing emotional intelligence helps men connect with their feelings, express themselves authentically, and foster deeper connections with others.

7. Preventive Health Screenings and Check-Ups:

- Preventive health screenings and regular check-ups are important for men's wellness, allowing early detection and management of potential health issues. Holistic approaches emphasize the importance of proactive health management, including regular physical exams, screenings for chronic conditions such as heart disease, diabetes, and cancer, and discussions with healthcare providers about lifestyle modifications and preventive strategies.

8. Holistic Therapies and Complementary Modalities:

- Holistic approaches to men's wellness incorporate a variety of complementary therapies and modalities to support overall health and well-being. These may include acupuncture, chiropractic care, massage therapy, naturopathic medicine, herbal remedies, energy healing, and mind-body practices such as biofeedback or hypnotherapy. Men are encouraged to explore and integrate these modalities as part of their holistic wellness plan, seeking out practitioners who specialize in men's health and well-being.

9. Environmental Awareness and Toxin Reduction:

   - Holistic approaches to men's wellness recognize the impact of environmental factors on health and well-being and emphasize the importance of environmental awareness and toxin reduction. Men are encouraged to minimize exposure to environmental toxins such as pollutants, pesticides, and harmful chemicals found in food, water, personal care products, and household items. Making informed choices about environmental health and adopting eco-friendly practices can support men's overall health and vitality.

10. Spiritual Exploration and Meaning-Making:

   - Holistic approaches to men's wellness acknowledge the importance of spiritual exploration and meaning-making as essential aspects of overall well-being. Men are encouraged to explore their spirituality, values, and beliefs, and to cultivate practices that foster a sense of purpose, connection, and inner peace. Whether through organized religion, meditation, nature connection, or other spiritual practices, men can tap into their spiritual dimension to enhance their sense of meaning and fulfillment in life.

Natural Approaches to Men's Reproductive Health

Natural approaches to men's reproductive health focus on supporting overall well-being, hormonal balance, and fertility through lifestyle modifications, nutrition, and targeted supplements. These approaches aim to optimize male reproductive function, sperm quality, and fertility potential while minimizing exposure to environmental toxins and supporting overall health and vitality. Here are key natural approaches to men's reproductive health:

1. Nutrition for Male Fertility:

- A nutrient-rich diet is essential for supporting male reproductive health and fertility. Men are encouraged to consume a balanced diet rich in fruits, vegetables, whole grains, lean proteins, healthy fats, and antioxidants. Specific nutrients such as zinc, selenium, vitamin C, vitamin E, folate, and omega-3 fatty acids play important roles in sperm production, motility, and morphology. Foods such as oysters, pumpkin seeds, spinach, berries, nuts, and fatty fish can be beneficial for male fertility.

2. Supplements for Male Fertility:
- Certain supplements may support male reproductive health and fertility by providing targeted nutrients that support sperm production, motility, and quality. These may include:
    - **Zinc:** Supports testosterone production and sperm quality.
    - **Selenium:** Enhances sperm motility and antioxidant defense.
    - **Coenzyme Q10 (CoQ10):** Improves sperm motility and mitochondrial function.
    - **L-arginine:** Supports sperm production and blood flow to the reproductive organs.
    - **Folate:** Important for DNA synthesis and sperm quality.
    - **Omega-3 fatty acids:** Support sperm membrane integrity and overall health.
- It's essential to consult with a healthcare provider before starting any new supplements to ensure safety and appropriate dosing.

3. Lifestyle Modifications for Male Fertility:
- Several lifestyle factors can impact male fertility, including smoking, excessive alcohol consumption, drug use, obesity, and sedentary behavior. Men are encouraged to adopt healthy lifestyle habits such as quitting smoking, limiting alcohol intake, avoiding recreational drugs, achieving and maintaining a healthy weight, and engaging in regular physical activity. Avoiding exposure to environmental toxins such as pesticides, heavy metals, and endocrine-disrupting chemicals is also important for preserving reproductive health.

4. Stress Management and Emotional Well-Being:
- Chronic stress and psychological factors can negatively impact male fertility by affecting hormone levels, sperm quality, and sexual function. Men are encouraged to practice stress-reduction techniques

such as meditation, deep breathing, yoga, mindfulness, or relaxation exercises to promote emotional well-being and hormonal balance. Seeking support from a therapist or counselor can also be beneficial for managing stress and addressing any underlying emotional issues that may affect fertility.

5. **Sleep Hygiene and Restorative Sleep:**
   - Quality sleep is essential for hormonal balance, energy levels, and overall health, including male fertility. Men are encouraged to prioritize sleep hygiene practices such as maintaining a regular sleep schedule, creating a relaxing bedtime routine, optimizing their sleep environment, and avoiding stimulants such as caffeine and electronic devices before bedtime. Adequate restorative sleep supports testosterone production, sperm quality, and reproductive health.

6. **Regular Physical Activity and Exercise:**
   - Regular physical activity and exercise are important for maintaining a healthy weight, improving blood flow, and supporting overall well-being, including male fertility. Men are encouraged to engage in regular moderate-intensity exercise such as brisk walking, jogging, cycling, swimming, or strength training. However, excessive or intense exercise may negatively impact fertility, so it's essential to strike a balance and avoid overtraining.

7. **Holistic Approaches to Reproductive Health:**
   - Holistic modalities such as acupuncture, chiropractic care, massage therapy, and traditional Chinese medicine (TCM) may offer additional support for male reproductive health and fertility. These modalities aim to balance the body's energy flow, promote relaxation, and support overall health and vitality. Some men may also benefit from herbal remedies or dietary supplements prescribed by a qualified practitioner of TCM or naturopathic medicine to address specific fertility concerns.

8. **Regular Health Check-Ups and Screenings:**
   - Men are encouraged to schedule regular health check-ups and screenings with their healthcare provider to monitor their reproductive health, hormone levels, and overall well-being. Routine screenings for conditions such as low testosterone, thyroid disorders, and other underlying health issues can help identify and address potential

fertility concerns early on. Maintaining open communication with a healthcare provider allows men to address any concerns or questions they may have about their reproductive health and fertility.

Balancing Hormones Holistically

Balancing hormones holistically involves adopting lifestyle changes, nutrition strategies, and natural therapies to support optimal hormone levels and promote overall health and vitality in men. Hormonal balance is essential for various physiological functions, including metabolism, energy levels, mood regulation, libido, and reproductive health. Here are holistic approaches to balancing hormones in men:

1. **Nutrition for Hormonal Health:**
   - Consuming a balanced diet rich in whole foods can support hormonal balance in men. Focus on nutrient-dense foods such as fruits, vegetables, lean proteins, healthy fats, and whole grains.
   - Include foods rich in specific nutrients that support hormone production and metabolism, such as zinc (found in oysters, pumpkin seeds, and beef), magnesium (found in nuts, seeds, and leafy greens), vitamin D (found in fatty fish, fortified foods, and sunlight exposure), and omega-3 fatty acids (found in fatty fish, flaxseeds, and walnuts).
   - Avoid processed foods, sugary snacks, and refined carbohydrates, as they can disrupt blood sugar levels and hormone balance.

2. **Stress Management:**
   - Chronic stress can disrupt hormone balance by increasing cortisol levels and impacting other hormone pathways. Incorporate stress-reduction techniques such as meditation, deep breathing exercises, yoga, mindfulness practices, and regular physical activity to manage stress levels effectively.
   - Prioritize adequate sleep and rest to support the body's stress response and hormone regulation. Aim for 7-9 hours of quality sleep per night and establish a relaxing bedtime routine.

3. **Regular Exercise:**
   - Engage in regular physical activity and exercise to support hormone balance and overall health. Both aerobic exercise and strength training

can help regulate hormone levels, improve insulin sensitivity, and support metabolic function.

- Aim for at least 150 minutes of moderate-intensity aerobic exercise or 75 minutes of vigorous-intensity exercise per week, along with muscle-strengthening activities on two or more days per week.

4. Weight Management:

- Maintaining a healthy weight is crucial for hormone balance, as excess body fat, especially around the abdomen, can contribute to hormonal imbalances such as insulin resistance and elevated estrogen levels.

- Focus on adopting a balanced diet and regular exercise routine to achieve and maintain a healthy weight. Incorporate strength training exercises to build lean muscle mass, which can help support metabolic health and hormone balance.

5. Limit Exposure to Endocrine Disruptors:

- Endocrine-disrupting chemicals (EDCs) found in certain plastics, pesticides, personal care products, and environmental pollutants can interfere with hormone function and contribute to hormonal imbalances.

- Minimize exposure to EDCs by choosing organic produce, using glass or stainless steel containers for food storage and beverages, avoiding plastic containers with BPA or phthalates, and selecting natural and chemical-free personal care products.

6. Herbal and Nutritional Supplements:

- Certain herbs and nutritional supplements may support hormone balance and overall well-being in men. Consult with a healthcare provider or qualified practitioner before starting any new supplements, as individual needs may vary.

- Examples of supplements that may support hormone balance include adaptogenic herbs such as ashwagandha and rhodiola, omega-3 fatty acids, vitamin D, magnesium, and zinc.

7. Regular Health Check-Ups:

- Schedule regular health check-ups with a healthcare provider to monitor hormone levels, assess overall health, and address any concerns or symptoms of hormonal imbalance.

- Consider hormone testing, such as measuring testosterone, cortisol, thyroid hormones, and other relevant markers, to gain insight into hormone status and potential imbalances.

8. Mind-Body Therapies:
- Mind-body therapies such as acupuncture, massage therapy, and biofeedback may help support hormone balance by promoting relaxation, reducing stress levels, and supporting overall well-being.
- Explore holistic modalities that focus on restoring balance and harmony in the body-mind connection to support hormone balance and overall health.

Mind-Body Practices for Stress Reduction

Mind-body practices offer effective techniques for stress reduction, promoting overall well-being and resilience in men. These practices help cultivate awareness of the mind-body connection, enabling individuals to manage stress more effectively and enhance their ability to cope with life's challenges. Here are several mind-body practices that can aid in stress reduction for men:

1. Meditation:
- Meditation involves focusing the mind on a particular object, thought, or activity to cultivate awareness and inner peace. Practices such as mindfulness meditation, loving-kindness meditation, and body scan meditation can help men reduce stress, promote relaxation, and enhance mental clarity.
- Men can start with short meditation sessions, gradually increasing the duration as they become more comfortable with the practice. Even just a few minutes of meditation each day can yield significant benefits for stress reduction and overall well-being.

2. Deep Breathing Exercises:
- Deep breathing exercises, such as diaphragmatic breathing or belly breathing, can help activate the body's relaxation response, reducing stress levels and promoting a sense of calm. By focusing on slow, deep breaths, men can release tension in the body and quiet the mind, creating a greater sense of ease and relaxation.

- Encourage men to practice deep breathing exercises throughout the day, especially during moments of stress or tension. Taking a few deep breaths before important meetings, during traffic jams, or before bedtime can help alleviate stress and promote a sense of inner peace.

3. Progressive Muscle Relaxation (PMR):

- PMR is a relaxation technique that involves tensing and then relaxing different muscle groups in the body, systematically releasing physical tension and promoting relaxation. Men can practice PMR by sequentially tensing and relaxing each muscle group, starting from the toes and working their way up to the head.

- PMR can be particularly effective for men who carry tension in their bodies or experience physical symptoms of stress, such as muscle stiffness or headaches. Regular practice can help men become more attuned to their bodies and better able to release tension when needed.

4. Yoga:

- Yoga combines physical postures, breathwork, and mindfulness practices to promote relaxation, flexibility, and inner peace. Men can benefit from practicing yoga regularly to reduce stress, increase body awareness, and cultivate a sense of balance and well-being.

- Encourage men to explore different styles of yoga, such as hatha, vinyasa, or yin yoga, to find a practice that resonates with them. Attending yoga classes or following online yoga videos can provide structure and guidance for those new to the practice.

5. Tai Chi and Qigong:

- Tai Chi and Qigong are gentle mind-body practices that involve slow, flowing movements, coordinated with deep breathing and mindfulness techniques. These ancient Chinese practices promote relaxation, balance, and vitality, making them ideal for stress reduction and overall well-being.

- Men can benefit from practicing Tai Chi or Qigong regularly to improve posture, enhance flexibility, and calm the mind. These practices are suitable for individuals of all ages and fitness levels, making them accessible options for stress reduction.

6. Guided Imagery and Visualization:

- Guided imagery and visualization involve using mental imagery to create a sense of relaxation, calmness, and well-being. Men can practice guided imagery by imagining peaceful scenes, such as a tranquil beach or serene forest, and engaging their senses to create a vivid mental experience.

- Guided imagery can be practiced independently or with the guidance of audio recordings or meditation apps. This practice can help men reduce stress, enhance mood, and improve their ability to cope with challenging situations.

Promoting Cardiovascular and Prostate Health

Promoting cardiovascular and prostate health is crucial for men's overall well-being and longevity. Adopting holistic approaches can address various factors that contribute to these aspects of men's health, including lifestyle modifications, dietary choices, stress management, and regular health screenings. Here's a comprehensive guide to promoting cardiovascular and prostate health holistically:

Cardiovascular Health:

1. Heart-Healthy Diet:
- Emphasize a diet rich in fruits, vegetables, whole grains, lean proteins (such as fish, poultry, legumes, and nuts), and healthy fats (such as olive oil and avocado).
- Reduce intake of processed foods, sugary beverages, saturated and trans fats, and excessive salt.
- Incorporate foods high in omega-3 fatty acids (such as fatty fish, flaxseeds, and walnuts) to support heart health and reduce inflammation.

2. Regular Exercise:
- Engage in regular physical activity, including aerobic exercises (such as brisk walking, jogging, cycling, or swimming) and strength training.
- Aim for at least 150 minutes of moderate-intensity aerobic activity or 75 minutes of vigorous-intensity aerobic activity per week, along with muscle-strengthening activities on two or more days per week.

3. Stress Management:

- Practice stress-reduction techniques such as deep breathing, meditation, yoga, tai chi, or mindfulness to lower stress levels and promote cardiovascular health.
- Ensure adequate rest and prioritize sleep hygiene practices to support overall well-being and stress management.

4. Maintain a Healthy Weight:

- Achieve and maintain a healthy weight through a balanced diet and regular exercise.
- Excess body weight, especially around the abdomen, increases the risk of cardiovascular disease, diabetes, and other health conditions.

5. Limit Alcohol and Avoid Smoking:

- Limit alcohol intake and avoid excessive consumption, as alcohol can contribute to high blood pressure and other cardiovascular risk factors.
- Quit smoking and avoid exposure to secondhand smoke, as smoking damages blood vessels and increases the risk of heart disease.

6. Regular Health Screenings:

- Schedule regular health check-ups with a healthcare provider to monitor blood pressure, cholesterol levels, and other cardiovascular risk factors.
- Discuss any concerns or symptoms with a healthcare provider and follow recommended screening guidelines for early detection and management of cardiovascular disease.

Prostate Health:

1. Prostate-Friendly Diet:

- Include foods rich in antioxidants, vitamins, minerals, and phytochemicals, such as fruits, vegetables, legumes, whole grains, nuts, seeds, and healthy fats.
- Consume foods high in omega-3 fatty acids (such as fatty fish) and lycopene (found in tomatoes and tomato products) to support prostate health.

2. Regular Physical Activity:

- Engage in regular exercise to support overall health and reduce the risk of prostate problems.
- Aim for at least 150 minutes of moderate-intensity aerobic activity or 75 minutes of vigorous-intensity aerobic activity per week, along with muscle-strengthening activities on two or more days per week.

3. Maintain a Healthy Weight:
- Maintain a healthy weight through a balanced diet and regular exercise, as obesity is associated with an increased risk of prostate cancer and other prostate issues.

4. Limit Red Meat and Dairy Products:
- Limit consumption of red meat and high-fat dairy products, as these may increase the risk of prostate cancer and other prostate problems.

5. Stay Hydrated and Limit Alcohol:
- Drink plenty of water and stay hydrated to support urinary and prostate health.
- Limit alcohol intake, as excessive alcohol consumption may increase the risk of prostate issues.

6. Regular Prostate Screenings:
- Discuss prostate health with a healthcare provider and follow recommended screening guidelines for prostate cancer, especially for men over 50 years old or those at higher risk.
- Screening tests may include a prostate-specific antigen (PSA) blood test, digital rectal exam (DRE), and other diagnostic tests as recommended by a healthcare provider.

Chapter 14
Holistic Approaches to Aging

Nurturing Holistic Health in the Aging Process

Nurturing holistic health during the aging process involves embracing a comprehensive approach that addresses the physical, mental, emotional, and spiritual aspects of well-being. By adopting holistic practices, individuals can optimize their health, vitality, and quality of life as they age. Here are key strategies for nurturing holistic health in the aging process:

1. Maintain a Balanced Diet:
- Consume a nutrient-rich diet that includes a variety of fruits, vegetables, whole grains, lean proteins, and healthy fats.
- Prioritize foods rich in antioxidants, vitamins, and minerals to support overall health and reduce the risk of age-related diseases.
- Stay hydrated by drinking an adequate amount of water and limit the intake of processed foods, sugary snacks, and excessive salt.

2. Stay Active:
- Engage in regular physical activity and exercise to maintain strength, flexibility, and cardiovascular health.
- Incorporate a combination of aerobic exercises, strength training, balance exercises, and flexibility exercises into your routine.
- Choose activities that you enjoy and can sustain over time, such as walking, swimming, yoga, tai chi, or dancing.

3. Prioritize Sleep and Rest:
- Ensure you get enough restorative sleep each night to support physical and mental well-being.
- Maintain a consistent sleep schedule, create a relaxing bedtime routine, and optimize your sleep environment for restful sleep.
- Practice relaxation techniques such as deep breathing, meditation, or gentle stretching before bedtime to promote relaxation and improve sleep quality.

4. Manage Stress Effectively:
- Practice stress-reduction techniques such as mindfulness meditation, deep breathing exercises, progressive muscle relaxation, or guided imagery.

- Cultivate a positive outlook, engage in hobbies and activities that bring joy, and maintain supportive social connections.
- Seek professional support if you're struggling with chronic stress, anxiety, or depression, and explore holistic therapies such as counseling, psychotherapy, or holistic healing modalities.

5. Cultivate Mental and Cognitive Well-Being:
- Keep your mind active and engaged by pursuing lifelong learning, challenging yourself with puzzles or brain games, and staying socially connected.
- Practice mindfulness and cognitive exercises to enhance cognitive function, memory, and mental clarity.
- Stay mentally stimulated by reading, writing, engaging in creative pursuits, or participating in stimulating conversations.

6. Nurture Emotional Health:
- Acknowledge and express your emotions in a healthy way, whether through journaling, talking with a trusted friend or counselor, or engaging in creative outlets.
- Practice self-compassion, acceptance, and resilience in the face of life's challenges and transitions.
- Cultivate a sense of purpose, meaning, and gratitude by focusing on what brings fulfillment and joy in your life.

7. Embrace Spirituality and Connection:
- Explore your spirituality and cultivate a sense of connection with something greater than yourself, whether through religion, nature, community, or personal beliefs.
- Engage in practices that nurture your spiritual well-being, such as prayer, meditation, spending time in nature, or participating in meaningful rituals or ceremonies.
- Foster supportive relationships and connections with loved ones, friends, and community members to enhance your sense of belonging and purpose.

8. Stay Proactive with Preventive Healthcare:
- Schedule regular check-ups and screenings with healthcare providers to monitor your health and detect any potential issues early.

- Stay up-to-date with vaccinations, preventive screenings, and recommended health assessments for your age and risk factors.
- Advocate for your health and well-being by being informed, proactive, and engaged in your healthcare decisions.

Mind-Body Practices for Healthy Aging

Mind-body practices are instrumental in promoting healthy aging by fostering physical, mental, emotional, and spiritual well-being. These practices cultivate mindfulness, reduce stress, enhance cognitive function, and support overall vitality as individuals age. Here are several mind-body practices for healthy aging:

1. **Mindfulness Meditation:**
- Mindfulness meditation involves focusing attention on the present moment without judgment, cultivating awareness of thoughts, sensations, and emotions.
- Regular practice of mindfulness meditation can reduce stress, improve mood, enhance cognitive function, and promote emotional resilience.
- Seniors can start with short meditation sessions and gradually increase duration and frequency over time. Guided meditation apps or classes may be helpful for beginners.

2. **Yoga:**
- Yoga combines physical postures (asanas), breathwork (pranayama), and meditation to promote flexibility, strength, balance, and relaxation.
- Practicing yoga can alleviate stiffness, improve mobility, reduce pain, and enhance overall well-being in older adults.
- Seniors can explore gentle yoga styles such as Hatha, Yin, or Chair Yoga, adapting poses to accommodate individual needs and limitations.

3. **Tai Chi and Qigong:**
- Tai Chi and Qigong are gentle mind-body practices originating from Chinese martial arts, characterized by slow, flowing movements and deep breathing.

- These practices improve balance, coordination, flexibility, and relaxation while reducing stress and promoting mental clarity.

- Seniors can benefit from regular Tai Chi or Qigong practice to maintain mobility, prevent falls, and enhance overall vitality.

4. Breathwork and Deep Breathing Exercises:

- Deep breathing exercises, such as diaphragmatic breathing or belly breathing, can induce relaxation, reduce stress, and enhance oxygenation.

- Seniors can practice deep breathing techniques throughout the day, particularly during moments of stress or tension, to promote calmness and well-being.

5. Progressive Muscle Relaxation (PMR):

- PMR involves systematically tensing and relaxing different muscle groups to release tension and promote relaxation.

- Seniors can practice PMR before bedtime to facilitate restful sleep or during the day to alleviate muscle stiffness and promote relaxation.

6. Guided Imagery and Visualization:

- Guided imagery involves creating mental images of peaceful and calming scenes to induce relaxation and reduce stress.

- Seniors can listen to guided imagery recordings or imagine serene landscapes, such as a tranquil beach or forest, to promote relaxation and well-being.

7. Creative Expression:

- Engaging in creative activities such as painting, drawing, writing, or playing music can stimulate the mind, foster self-expression, and promote emotional well-being.

- Seniors can explore hobbies and creative outlets that bring joy and fulfillment, nurturing their sense of purpose and vitality.

8. Nature Connection:

- Spending time in nature, whether through walking in parks, gardening, or enjoying outdoor activities, can promote relaxation, reduce stress, and enhance overall well-being.

- Seniors can prioritize outdoor time and connect with the natural world to nurture their spirit and sense of connection with the environment.

Nutrition and Lifestyle for Longevity

Nutrition and lifestyle play pivotal roles in promoting longevity and overall well-being as individuals age. Adopting holistic approaches to nutrition and lifestyle can support healthy aging by nourishing the body, enhancing vitality, and reducing the risk of chronic diseases. Here's a comprehensive guide to nutrition and lifestyle for longevity:

Nutrition for Longevity:

1. **Plant-Based Diet:**
   - Emphasize a predominantly plant-based diet rich in fruits, vegetables, whole grains, legumes, nuts, and seeds.
   - Plant-based diets are abundant in vitamins, minerals, antioxidants, and phytonutrients, which promote cellular health, reduce inflammation, and support overall well-being.

2. **Healthy Fats:**
   - Include sources of healthy fats such as avocados, nuts, seeds, olive oil, and fatty fish (e.g., salmon, mackerel) in your diet.
   - Omega-3 fatty acids found in fatty fish, flaxseeds, and walnuts have anti-inflammatory properties and support heart health and cognitive function.

3. **Lean Proteins:**
   - Choose lean protein sources such as poultry, fish, tofu, tempeh, legumes, and low-fat dairy products.
   - Protein is essential for muscle maintenance, immune function, and tissue repair, particularly as individuals age.

4. **Moderate Caloric Intake:**
   - Practice mindful eating and portion control to maintain a healthy weight and prevent overeating.

- Avoid excessive calorie consumption, as caloric restriction has been associated with increased longevity and reduced risk of age-related diseases.

5. Hydration:
- Stay adequately hydrated by drinking water throughout the day.
- Proper hydration supports digestion, cognitive function, joint health, and overall cellular function.

6. Antioxidant-Rich Foods:
- Include antioxidant-rich foods such as berries, dark leafy greens, cruciferous vegetables, and colorful fruits and vegetables in your diet.
- Antioxidants protect cells from oxidative stress and inflammation, helping to reduce the risk of chronic diseases associated with aging.

Lifestyle for Longevity:

1. Regular Physical Activity:
- Engage in regular exercise to maintain cardiovascular health, muscle strength, flexibility, and balance.
- Aim for at least 150 minutes of moderate-intensity aerobic activity or 75 minutes of vigorous-intensity aerobic activity per week, along with muscle-strengthening activities on two or more days per week.

2. Stress Management:
- Practice stress-reduction techniques such as mindfulness meditation, deep breathing exercises, yoga, tai chi, or progressive muscle relaxation.
- Chronic stress contributes to inflammation, oxidative stress, and accelerated aging, so it's essential to prioritize stress management techniques.

3. Quality Sleep:
- Prioritize restorative sleep by maintaining a consistent sleep schedule, creating a relaxing bedtime routine, and optimizing your sleep environment.
- Aim for 7-9 hours of quality sleep per night to support cognitive function, immune health, and overall well-being.

4. **Social Connections:**
   - Maintain strong social connections and cultivate meaningful relationships with family, friends, and community members.
   - Social engagement is associated with improved mental health, emotional well-being, and longevity.

5. **Cognitive Stimulation:**
   - Stay mentally active by engaging in lifelong learning, challenging puzzles, brain games, reading, or participating in stimulating conversations.
   - Cognitive stimulation promotes brain health, memory retention, and cognitive function as individuals age.

6. **Purpose and Meaning:**
   - Cultivate a sense of purpose, meaning, and fulfillment by pursuing activities, hobbies, and interests that bring joy and satisfaction.
   - Having a sense of purpose is associated with greater resilience, longevity, and overall well-being.

Holistic Perspectives on Cognitive Health

Holistic perspectives on cognitive health encompass a comprehensive approach to maintaining and enhancing cognitive function throughout the aging process. These perspectives recognize the interconnectedness of various factors, including lifestyle, nutrition, mental stimulation, social engagement, and emotional well-being, in promoting optimal brain health and cognitive vitality. Here's a guide to holistic approaches to cognitive health:

Lifestyle Factors:

1. **Regular Physical Activity:**
   - Engage in regular aerobic exercise, strength training, and balance exercises to support brain health and cognitive function.
   - Exercise increases blood flow to the brain, promotes neuroplasticity, and stimulates the production of brain-derived neurotrophic factor (BDNF), a protein that supports the growth and survival of brain cells.

2. Healthy Diet:
  - Follow a Mediterranean-style diet rich in fruits, vegetables, whole grains, healthy fats (such as olive oil and nuts), and lean proteins (such as fish and poultry).
  - Antioxidant-rich foods, omega-3 fatty acids, and polyphenols found in plant-based foods protect against oxidative stress and inflammation, promoting brain health.

3. Quality Sleep:
  - Prioritize restorative sleep by maintaining a regular sleep schedule, creating a conducive sleep environment, and practicing relaxation techniques before bedtime.
  - Adequate sleep is essential for memory consolidation, cognitive function, and overall brain health.

4. Stress Management:
  - Practice stress-reduction techniques such as mindfulness meditation, deep breathing exercises, yoga, or tai chi to lower stress levels and support brain health.
  - Chronic stress can negatively impact cognitive function and increase the risk of cognitive decline and neurodegenerative diseases.

5. Social Engagement:
  - Stay socially connected and maintain meaningful relationships with friends, family, and community members.
  - Social interaction stimulates cognitive function, reduces the risk of cognitive decline, and promotes emotional well-being.

Mental Stimulation:

1. Lifelong Learning:
  - Engage in intellectually stimulating activities such as reading, puzzles, crossword puzzles, learning a new language, or taking up a hobby or skill.
  - Cognitive stimulation promotes neuroplasticity, strengthens neural connections, and preserves cognitive function as individuals age.

2. Brain Training:

- Use brain training programs or apps designed to challenge memory, attention, and problem-solving skills.
- While research on the efficacy of brain training is mixed, engaging in cognitively stimulating activities can still be beneficial for cognitive health.

Emotional and Spiritual Well-Being:

1. Emotional Resilience:
- Cultivate emotional resilience through mindfulness practices, self-compassion, and acceptance of life's challenges.
- Emotional well-being supports cognitive function and helps individuals cope with stress and adversity.

2. Spiritual Practices:
- Engage in spiritual practices such as meditation, prayer, or contemplation to foster inner peace, meaning, and purpose.
- Spirituality can provide a sense of connection, transcendence, and resilience, which contribute to overall well-being, including cognitive health.

Brain-Healthy Habits:

1. Brain-Boosting Nutrients:
- Incorporate foods rich in brain-boosting nutrients such as omega-3 fatty acids, antioxidants, vitamins, and minerals into your diet.
- Examples include fatty fish, walnuts, blueberries, spinach, broccoli, and dark chocolate.

2. Hydration:
- Stay adequately hydrated by drinking water throughout the day to support cognitive function and brain health.

3. Limit Alcohol and Avoid Smoking:
- Limit alcohol consumption and avoid smoking, as both can negatively impact cognitive function and increase the risk of cognitive decline.

Building Holistic Communities for Elderly Well-Being

Building holistic communities for elderly well-being involves creating supportive environments that address the physical, mental, emotional, social, and spiritual needs of older adults. These communities promote independence, dignity, and quality of life while fostering connections, purpose, and a sense of belonging. Here's how to create holistic communities for elderly well-being:

 Physical Environment:

1. **Accessible Design:**
   - Ensure that buildings and public spaces are designed with accessibility in mind, including wheelchair ramps, handrails, elevators, and wide doorways.
   - Create age-friendly environments that accommodate mobility challenges and promote safety and independence for older adults.

2. **Green Spaces:**
   - Incorporate gardens, parks, and outdoor seating areas into the community to provide opportunities for relaxation, socialization, and connection with nature.
   - Access to green spaces supports physical activity, reduces stress, and enhances overall well-being.

 Social Engagement:

1. **Community Centers:**
   - Establish community centers or gathering spaces where older adults can come together for social activities, events, and programs.
   - Offer a variety of activities such as exercise classes, art workshops, book clubs, cooking demonstrations, and cultural events to foster social connections and engagement.

2. **Intergenerational Programs:**

- Facilitate intergenerational programs that bring together older adults and younger generations for mutual learning, companionship, and support.
- Activities may include mentoring programs, volunteer opportunities, or joint projects with local schools or youth organizations.

Supportive Services:

1. **Health and Wellness Services:**
- Provide access to healthcare services, wellness programs, and preventive screenings within the community.
- Offer on-site clinics, health education workshops, fitness classes, and nutritional counseling to support holistic health and well-being.

2. **Caregiver Support:**
- Offer resources, respite services, and support groups for family caregivers who are caring for older adults within the community.
- Provide information, education, and assistance to help caregivers navigate the challenges of caregiving and maintain their own well-being.

Mental and Emotional Well-Being:

1. **Mental Health Services:**
- Offer counseling, therapy, and support groups for older adults dealing with mental health issues such as depression, anxiety, grief, or cognitive decline.
- Provide opportunities for mindfulness meditation, relaxation techniques, and stress management workshops to promote emotional well-being.

2. **Life Enrichment Programs:**
- Create opportunities for lifelong learning, creative expression, and personal growth through educational workshops, art classes, music therapy, and cultural enrichment activities.
- Empower older adults to pursue their interests, passions, and hobbies, fostering a sense of purpose and fulfillment.

Spiritual and Meaningful Engagement:

1. Spiritual Support:

   - Offer spiritual care services, chaplaincy programs, and opportunities for prayer, meditation, or spiritual reflection within the community.
   - Respect and honor diverse spiritual and religious beliefs, providing inclusive spaces for individuals to explore and express their spirituality.

2. Meaningful Activities:

   - Encourage participation in meaningful activities that align with individual values, beliefs, and interests.
   - Provide opportunities for volunteering, community service, and contributing to the greater good, fostering a sense of purpose and connection.

Technology and Innovation:

1. Digital Inclusion:

   - Promote digital literacy and provide access to technology resources such as computers, tablets, and internet connectivity to bridge the digital divide among older adults.
   - Offer technology training, virtual communication tools, and telehealth services to enhance access to information, services, and social connections.

Community Engagement and Empowerment:

1. Resident Involvement:

   - Foster resident involvement and empowerment by soliciting feedback, ideas, and contributions from older adults in shaping community programs, policies, and initiatives.
   - Create opportunities for older adults to be actively engaged in decision-making, leadership roles, and community governance.

2. Peer Support Networks:

   - Facilitate peer support networks and buddy systems where older adults can connect with one another, share experiences, and provide mutual support.

- Peer support fosters a sense of camaraderie, belonging, and resilience among community members.

Chapter 15
Holistic Parenting

Holistic Approaches to Pregnancy

Holistic approaches to pregnancy focus on nurturing the physical, emotional, and spiritual well-being of both the expectant mother and her baby. These approaches encompass a variety of practices that support a healthy pregnancy, promote optimal fetal development, and prepare the mother for childbirth and postpartum recovery. Here are some holistic approaches to pregnancy:

Nutrition and Diet:

1. Whole Foods Diet:
   - Emphasize a balanced diet rich in whole, nutrient-dense foods such as fruits, vegetables, whole grains, lean proteins, and healthy fats.
   - Choose organic and locally sourced foods when possible to minimize exposure to pesticides and toxins.

2. Hydration:
   - Drink plenty of water throughout the day to stay hydrated and support the body's physiological changes during pregnancy.
   - Herbal teas and coconut water can also provide hydration and additional nutrients.

3. Supplementation:
   - Take prenatal vitamins containing folic acid, iron, calcium, vitamin D, omega-3 fatty acids, and other essential nutrients to support fetal development and maternal health.
   - Consult with a healthcare provider or holistic practitioner to determine specific supplement needs based on individual health status.

Mind-Body Practices:

1. Prenatal Yoga and Meditation:
   - Practice prenatal yoga and meditation to reduce stress, alleviate discomfort, and promote relaxation during pregnancy.
   - These practices can also help expectant mothers connect with their bodies and bond with their babies.

2. Breathwork and Relaxation Techniques:

- Learn and practice deep breathing exercises, visualization, and progressive muscle relaxation to manage anxiety, fear, and pain during pregnancy and childbirth.

- Hypnobirthing and mindfulness techniques can also be beneficial for promoting a calm and positive birth experience.

Emotional Support:

1. Holistic Counseling and Therapy:

- Seek support from holistic counselors or therapists who specialize in pregnancy-related issues, childbirth preparation, and postpartum adjustment.

- Addressing emotional concerns and psychological stressors can positively impact maternal and fetal well-being.

2. Community and Peer Support:

- Connect with other expectant mothers through prenatal yoga classes, support groups, online forums, and community events.

- Sharing experiences, exchanging information, and receiving support from peers can help alleviate feelings of isolation and anxiety.

Bodywork and Movement:

1. Chiropractic Care:

- Consider chiropractic adjustments to address musculoskeletal issues, alleviate back pain, and promote optimal pelvic alignment for childbirth.

- Prenatal chiropractic care can also support overall comfort and well-being during pregnancy.

2. Massage Therapy:

- Receive regular prenatal massage therapy to reduce muscle tension, improve circulation, and alleviate discomfort associated with pregnancy.

- Massage can also promote relaxation, stress reduction, and emotional well-being.

Traditional and Complementary Therapies:

1. Acupuncture and Traditional Chinese Medicine (TCM):
   - Explore acupuncture and TCM modalities such as acupressure, herbal medicine, and dietary therapy to address common pregnancy symptoms and promote balance within the body.
   - These therapies may help alleviate nausea, fatigue, insomnia, and other pregnancy-related issues.

2. Homeopathy and Naturopathy:
   - Consult with qualified homeopaths or naturopathic doctors for personalized recommendations on natural remedies, dietary supplements, and lifestyle modifications to support a healthy pregnancy.
   - Homeopathic remedies and naturopathic therapies can complement conventional prenatal care and promote holistic well-being.

Environmental Health:

1. Toxin Avoidance:
   - Minimize exposure to environmental toxins, pollutants, and harmful chemicals by choosing natural and non-toxic personal care products, household cleaners, and food containers.
   - Create a safe and healthy home environment for the expectant mother and her baby.

2. Mindful Living:
   - Practice mindful living by being conscious of the impact of daily choices on health and well-being.
   - Prioritize natural and sustainable practices that support ecological balance and contribute to a healthy environment for future generations.

Holistic Childbirth Education:

1. Childbirth Classes:
   - Attend comprehensive childbirth education classes that incorporate holistic approaches to childbirth, including natural pain management techniques, labor support strategies, and informed decision-making.
   - Learn about the physiological process of birth, stages of labor, and coping mechanisms for labor and delivery.

2. **Birth Planning:**
   - Create a birth plan that reflects your preferences and values regarding childbirth interventions, pain management options, and postpartum care.
   - Collaborate with healthcare providers who support holistic and evidence-based maternity care practices.

Natural Parenting Practices

Natural parenting practices, also known as attachment parenting or instinctive parenting, prioritize nurturing the parent-child bond, meeting the child's needs holistically, and supporting their development in alignment with nature's rhythms. These practices emphasize responsiveness, connection, and gentle guidance, recognizing the importance of biological and emotional instincts in parenting. Here are some key principles of natural parenting:

Breastfeeding:

1. **Breastfeeding On-Demand:**
   - Respond to the baby's hunger cues and feed on demand, promoting a responsive feeding approach that fosters trust and security.
   - Breast milk provides optimal nutrition, immune support, and emotional bonding between parent and child.

2. **Extended Breastfeeding:**
   - Support extended breastfeeding beyond infancy, acknowledging the continued nutritional and emotional benefits for both the child and the parent.
   - Respect the child's natural weaning process and individual readiness for transitioning to solid foods.

Co-Sleeping and Bed-Sharing:

1. **Safe Co-Sleeping Practices:**

- Practice safe co-sleeping by following guidelines to reduce the risk of Sudden Infant Death Syndrome (SIDS) and ensure a safe sleep environment.
- Co-sleeping promotes secure attachment, facilitates nighttime breastfeeding, and enhances parental responsiveness to the child's needs.

2. Bed-Sharing:

- Consider bed-sharing as a natural extension of co-sleeping, allowing for increased physical proximity and emotional connection between parent and child.
- Follow safety guidelines to minimize the risk of accidents and ensure a safe sleeping environment for everyone.

Babywearing:

1. Skin-to-Skin Contact:

- Utilize baby carriers, slings, wraps, or kangaroo care to keep the baby close and maintain skin-to-skin contact, promoting bonding, comfort, and emotional regulation.
- Babywearing allows parents to attend to daily activities while nurturing their child's need for closeness and security.

Responsive Parenting:

1. Attachment Parenting Principles:

- Practice responsive parenting by sensitively attuning to the child's cues, needs, and emotions, fostering a secure attachment bond.
- Respond promptly to the child's cries, provide comfort and reassurance, and prioritize connection and emotional support.

Gentle Discipline:

1. Positive Discipline:

- Use positive discipline techniques such as redirection, modeling, and setting clear boundaries with empathy and understanding.
- Avoid punitive measures and focus on guiding the child's behavior through respectful communication and mutual cooperation.

Natural Health and Wellness:

1. Holistic Healthcare:
   - Prioritize natural approaches to healthcare, including preventive measures, natural remedies, and integrative therapies that support the child's physical, emotional, and mental well-being.
   - Consult with holistic healthcare providers, such as naturopathic doctors or holistic pediatricians, who emphasize a whole-person approach to wellness.

Respectful Parenting:

1. Respect for the Child's Autonomy:
   - Honor the child's autonomy, preferences, and developmental stage by involving them in decision-making and respecting their choices whenever possible.
   - Recognize the child as a unique individual with their own thoughts, feelings, and needs.

Mindful Parenting:

1. Presence and Mindfulness:
   - Practice mindfulness and presence in parenting, cultivating awareness of the present moment and tuning into the child's cues, needs, and emotions.
   - Mindful parenting fosters a deeper connection, emotional attunement, and mutual understanding between parent and child.

Eco-Friendly Practices:

1. Natural and Sustainable Living:
   - Embrace eco-friendly practices such as using organic and non-toxic products, reducing waste, and minimizing environmental impact on the planet.
   - Raise awareness about environmental stewardship and model sustainable behaviors for future generations.

Natural parenting practices emphasize nurturing the parent-child relationship, promoting emotional security, and supporting the child's holistic development in harmony with nature's principles. These practices prioritize connection, responsiveness, and respect for the child's innate needs and individuality.

Mind-Body Wellness for New Parents

Mind-body wellness for new parents involves nurturing physical, mental, and emotional well-being while navigating the transformative journey of parenthood. It encompasses practices that promote self-care, stress reduction, emotional balance, and resilience during this period of significant change and adjustment. Here are some holistic strategies for promoting mind-body wellness for new parents:

Physical Well-Being:

1. **Prioritize Rest and Sleep:**
   - Get adequate rest and sleep whenever possible, even if it means taking short naps throughout the day.
   - Establish a bedtime routine to promote relaxation and improve sleep quality.

2. **Nutritious Eating Habits:**
   - Maintain a balanced diet with nutrient-rich foods to support energy levels, physical recovery, and overall well-being.
   - Plan and prepare simple, nourishing meals and snacks that are easy to grab and eat on-the-go.

3. **Stay Hydrated:**
   - Drink plenty of water throughout the day to stay hydrated, especially if breastfeeding or experiencing postpartum changes.
   - Limit caffeine and sugary beverages, opting for water, herbal teas, and natural fruit juices instead.

4. **Gentle Movement:**
   - Engage in gentle movement activities such as walking, stretching, or postnatal yoga to promote circulation, flexibility, and physical comfort.

- Listen to your body and avoid strenuous exercise until cleared by a healthcare provider.

Mental and Emotional Well-Being:

1. Practice Self-Compassion:
- Be gentle and patient with yourself as you navigate the challenges and joys of parenthood.
- Recognize and validate your feelings, knowing that it's normal to experience a range of emotions during this time.

2. Mindfulness and Stress Reduction:
- Incorporate mindfulness practices such as deep breathing, meditation, or mindful parenting techniques to reduce stress and cultivate presence.
- Take breaks throughout the day to pause, breathe, and center yourself, especially during moments of overwhelm.

3. Seek Support:
- Reach out to friends, family members, or support groups for emotional support, practical assistance, and validation of your experiences.
- Consider joining parenting classes, online communities, or peer support groups to connect with other new parents and share resources.

4. Set Realistic Expectations:
- Adjust your expectations and priorities to align with the realities of new parenthood.
- Focus on small, achievable goals and celebrate your accomplishments, no matter how minor they may seem.

Relationship Wellness:

1. Maintain Connection with Your Partner:
- Make time for meaningful connection with your partner, even amidst the demands of parenting.
- Schedule regular date nights, communicate openly, and express appreciation for each other's efforts.

2. Co-Parenting Strategies:

- Establish clear communication and shared responsibilities with your co-parent to ensure a harmonious parenting partnership.
- Collaborate on decision-making, parenting techniques, and household tasks to lighten the load and promote mutual support.

3. Bonding with Your Baby:

- Prioritize bonding time with your baby through skin-to-skin contact, cuddling, babywearing, and responsive caregiving.
- Create daily rituals and routines that strengthen the parent-child bond and promote attachment.

Time for Self-Care:

1. Schedule Me-Time:

- Carve out time for self-care activities that nourish your body, mind, and soul.
- Whether it's a bubble bath, reading a book, or pursuing a hobby, prioritize activities that replenish your energy and bring you joy.

2. Delegate and Ask for Help:

- Delegate tasks and responsibilities to family members, friends, or hired help when needed.
- Don't hesitate to ask for assistance with childcare, household chores, or errands to lighten your workload and create space for self-care.

3. Practice Boundaries:

- Set boundaries around your time, energy, and commitments to avoid burnout and overwhelm.
- Learn to say no to non-essential obligations and prioritize activities that align with your values and well-being.

Professional Support:

1. Access Professional Resources:

- Seek guidance from healthcare providers, lactation consultants, therapists, or parenting coaches if you're struggling with physical or emotional challenges.

- Don't hesitate to reach out for professional support when needed, as early intervention can help prevent issues from escalating.

Holistic Child Development

Holistic child development encompasses nurturing the physical, emotional, cognitive, social, and spiritual aspects of a child's growth and well-being. It recognizes the interconnectedness of these domains and emphasizes creating supportive environments that foster holistic development. Here are key principles and practices for holistic child development:

 Physical Well-Being:

1. Healthy Nutrition:
   - Provide a balanced diet rich in fruits, vegetables, whole grains, lean proteins, and healthy fats to support physical growth, brain development, and overall health.
   - Model healthy eating habits and involve children in meal planning and preparation to instill lifelong healthy habits.

2. Regular Physical Activity:
   - Encourage regular exercise and active play to promote physical fitness, coordination, and motor skills development.
   - Provide opportunities for outdoor play, sports activities, and movement-based games to support gross and fine motor development.

3. Adequate Rest and Sleep:
   - Ensure children get sufficient rest and sleep according to their age and individual needs.
   - Establish consistent bedtime routines, create a calm sleep environment, and prioritize sleep hygiene practices to support quality sleep.

 Emotional Well-Being:

1. Emotional Awareness and Expression:

- Foster emotional intelligence by teaching children to recognize, label, and express their emotions in healthy ways.
- Create a safe and supportive environment where children feel comfortable sharing their feelings and experiences without judgment.

2. Attachment and Bonding:

- Cultivate secure attachments between caregivers and children through responsive, nurturing, and sensitive caregiving practices.
- Promote bonding through physical affection, positive interactions, and attentive listening, strengthening the parent-child relationship.

3. Emotion Regulation Skills:

- Teach children effective emotion regulation strategies such as deep breathing, mindfulness, and problem-solving techniques to manage stress and cope with difficult emotions.
- Model self-regulation skills and provide guidance and support as children learn to navigate their emotions.

Cognitive Development:

1. Stimulating Environment:

- Create a rich and stimulating environment that encourages exploration, curiosity, and intellectual engagement.
- Provide age-appropriate toys, books, puzzles, and activities that stimulate cognitive development and problem-solving skills.

2. Play-Based Learning:

- Emphasize play-based learning as a natural and effective way for children to learn, explore, and make sense of the world around them.
- Encourage imaginative play, creative expression, and hands-on exploration to foster cognitive, social, and emotional development.

3. Encourage Curiosity and Critical Thinking:

- Support children's natural curiosity by encouraging questions, exploration, and experimentation.
- Foster critical thinking skills by encouraging children to analyze, question, and evaluate information, fostering independence and autonomy.

Social Development:

1. Peer Interaction:
   - Provide opportunities for positive peer interactions and socialization through playdates, group activities, and community events.
   - Teach children cooperation, empathy, and communication skills to navigate social relationships effectively.

2. Community Engagement:
   - Engage children in community service projects, volunteer activities, and cultural experiences to broaden their perspectives and foster a sense of social responsibility.
   - Model kindness, compassion, and respect for diversity, promoting empathy and understanding of others.

3. Conflict Resolution Skills:
   - Teach children constructive conflict resolution skills such as active listening, negotiation, and compromise to resolve conflicts peacefully.
   - Encourage open communication, empathy, and perspective-taking to promote positive peer relationships and social harmony.

Spiritual Well-Being:

1. Cultivate Inner Values and Beliefs:
   - Foster children's spiritual development by exploring and discussing values, beliefs, and existential questions in age-appropriate ways.
   - Encourage reflection, gratitude, and mindfulness practices that nurture a sense of inner peace, purpose, and connection to something greater than oneself.

2. Connection with Nature and the Universe:
   - Foster children's connection with nature by spending time outdoors, exploring natural environments, and appreciating the beauty and wonder of the natural world.
   - Encourage awe, wonder, and reverence for the interconnectedness of all living beings and the universe.

Holistic Parenting Practices:

1. **Responsive and Attuned Caregiving:**
   - Practice responsive and attuned caregiving that meets children's physical, emotional, and developmental needs with sensitivity and compassion.
   - Create a nurturing and supportive home environment where children feel loved, valued, and respected for who they are.

2. **Balanced Approach to Discipline:**
   - Use a balanced approach to discipline that emphasizes positive reinforcement, clear boundaries, and constructive guidance rather than punitive measures.
   - Teach children self-discipline, self-regulation, and responsibility through positive reinforcement, modeling, and consistent expectations.

3. **Lifelong Learning and Growth:**
   - Cultivate a culture of lifelong learning and growth within the family, promoting curiosity, resilience, and a growth mindset.
   - Encourage children to embrace challenges, learn from failures, and pursue their interests and passions with enthusiasm and perseverance.

Creating Holistic Environments for Children

Creating holistic environments for children involves designing spaces that support their physical, emotional, cognitive, social, and spiritual well-being. These environments should promote a sense of safety, connection, and harmony, fostering holistic development and overall wellness. Here are key elements to consider when creating holistic environments for children:

Physical Environment:

1. **Safe and Nurturing Spaces:**
   - Ensure that the physical environment is safe, clean, and free from hazards to promote children's physical health and safety.
   - Design spaces that are warm, inviting, and aesthetically pleasing, incorporating natural elements, soft textures, and soothing colors.

2. Outdoor Access:

   - Provide access to outdoor spaces such as gardens, playgrounds, and nature trails to encourage exploration, physical activity, and connection with nature.
   - Create outdoor play areas that offer opportunities for imaginative play, sensory exploration, and gross motor development.

3. Healthy Materials and Furnishings:

   - Choose non-toxic, eco-friendly materials and furnishings that support indoor air quality and minimize exposure to harmful chemicals.
   - Opt for natural materials such as wood, cotton, wool, and bamboo for furniture, toys, and decor items whenever possible.

Emotional Environment:

1. Warm and Responsive Relationships:

   - Cultivate warm, responsive, and nurturing relationships between caregivers and children to create a supportive emotional environment.
   - Foster a sense of security and trust through attentive listening, affectionate interactions, and consistent caregiving routines.

2. Comforting Spaces for Emotional Regulation:

   - Design cozy and comforting spaces within the environment where children can retreat to regulate their emotions and find solace during times of distress.
   - Provide soft pillows, blankets, stuffed animals, and calming sensory materials to support emotional self-regulation and relaxation.

3. Art and Creative Expression:

   - Incorporate opportunities for creative expression and artistic activities such as drawing, painting, sculpting, and crafting into the environment.
   - Display children's artwork and creations prominently to celebrate their creativity, self-expression, and individuality.

Cognitive Environment:

1. Stimulating Learning Materials:

- Offer a variety of age-appropriate learning materials, books, puzzles, and educational toys that stimulate curiosity, exploration, and cognitive development.
- Rotate materials regularly to keep the environment fresh and engaging, encouraging children to discover new interests and pursue independent exploration.

2. Learning Centers and Zones:

- Create designated learning centers or zones within the environment for different types of play and learning experiences, such as a reading corner, art studio, science lab, or dramatic play area.
- Provide opportunities for hands-on exploration, experimentation, and discovery in each learning center to support diverse learning styles and interests.

3. Flexible and Open-ended Play Spaces:

- Design flexible and open-ended play spaces that allow children to engage in unstructured, child-directed play and experimentation.
- Provide loose parts, open-ended materials, and multi-purpose play equipment that encourage creativity, problem-solving, and imaginative play.

Social Environment:

1. Collaborative and Cooperative Play:

- Foster a culture of collaboration, cooperation, and inclusivity within the environment, encouraging children to work together, share resources, and solve problems collaboratively.
- Design group play areas and cooperative games that promote teamwork, communication, and social skills development.

2. Positive Peer Relationships:

- Create opportunities for positive peer interactions and socialization through group activities, cooperative play, and collaborative projects.
- Facilitate conflict resolution and teach children effective communication and problem-solving skills to navigate social relationships respectfully.

Spiritual Environment:

1. **Connection with Nature and Spirituality:**
   - Foster a sense of connection with nature and spirituality by incorporating natural elements, sacred symbols, and mindfulness practices into the environment.
   - Create outdoor nature corners, meditation spaces, or quiet reflection areas where children can connect with the natural world and explore their inner selves.

2. **Values and Ethics:**
   - Promote values such as kindness, compassion, empathy, and respect for all living beings within the environment.
   - Encourage discussions about ethical dilemmas, social justice issues, and global citizenship to cultivate children's moral reasoning and spiritual awareness.

Holistic Integration:

1. **Mindfulness and Wellness Practices:**
   - Integrate mindfulness, relaxation, and wellness practices into the daily routine, such as mindfulness exercises, guided imagery, yoga, or deep breathing exercises.
   - Create opportunities for children to practice mindfulness and self-care techniques to promote emotional resilience, stress reduction, and overall well-being.

2. **Connection with Community and Culture:**
   - Foster a sense of connection with the broader community and diverse cultural traditions by celebrating holidays, festivals, and cultural events within the environment.
   - Invite guest speakers, cultural performers, or community members to share their experiences, stories, and talents with the children.

Chapter 16
Holistic Education and Learning

Holistic Perspectives on Education

Holistic education encompasses a comprehensive approach to learning that addresses the diverse needs of learners and nurtures their physical, emotional, cognitive, social, and spiritual well-being. It goes beyond traditional academic instruction to promote holistic development and empower individuals to thrive in all aspects of their lives. Here are key holistic perspectives on education:

1. Whole-Person Approach:
  - Holistic education views learners as complex beings with interconnected physical, emotional, intellectual, social, and spiritual dimensions.
  - It recognizes the importance of addressing the needs of the whole person, not just academic achievement, in the educational process.

2. Inclusivity and Diversity:
  - Holistic education values and celebrates diversity in all its forms, including cultural, linguistic, socio-economic, and neurodiversity.
  - It promotes inclusive learning environments where all students feel valued, respected, and supported in their unique identities and abilities.

3. Experiential and Inquiry-Based Learning:
  - Holistic education emphasizes hands-on, experiential learning opportunities that engage learners in active exploration, discovery, and reflection.
  - It encourages inquiry-based approaches that stimulate curiosity, critical thinking, and problem-solving skills, fostering lifelong learners.

4. Emotional Intelligence and Well-Being:
  - Holistic education prioritizes the development of emotional intelligence and well-being alongside academic achievement.
  - It teaches students self-awareness, self-regulation, empathy, and interpersonal skills, empowering them to navigate their emotions and relationships effectively.

5. Relationship-Centered Learning:

- Holistic education values positive relationships between students, educators, families, and communities as foundational to learning and growth.
- It promotes collaborative learning environments where trust, respect, and empathy are cultivated, fostering a sense of belonging and connection.

6. Nature-Based and Environmental Education:
- Holistic education recognizes the importance of connecting with nature and integrating environmental education into the curriculum.
- It encourages outdoor learning experiences, ecological awareness, and sustainable practices that foster environmental stewardship and a sense of interconnectedness with the natural world.

7. Mindfulness and Contemplative Practices:
- Holistic education integrates mindfulness, meditation, and contemplative practices into the learning process to promote focus, presence, and inner peace.
- It teaches students stress reduction techniques, relaxation exercises, and mindfulness-based coping strategies to enhance well-being and academic performance.

8. Values and Ethical Education:
- Holistic education emphasizes the importance of values, ethics, and character development in shaping responsible global citizens.
- It fosters discussions about ethical dilemmas, social justice issues, and moral decision-making, empowering students to act with integrity and compassion.

9. Creative Expression and Arts Integration:
- Holistic education values the role of creativity, imagination, and artistic expression in learning and personal development.
- It integrates arts education, music, drama, visual arts, and creative writing into the curriculum to nurture self-expression, innovation, and cultural appreciation.

10. Lifelong Learning and Personal Growth:
- Holistic education instills a love of learning and a growth mindset that values curiosity, resilience, and continuous personal growth.

- It empowers students to take ownership of their learning journey, set goals, pursue their passions, and adapt to a rapidly changing world.

Integrating Mindfulness in Learning Environments

Integrating mindfulness into learning environments is an effective way to promote holistic development, emotional well-being, and academic success among students. Mindfulness practices help cultivate present moment awareness, focus, self-regulation, and stress reduction skills, which are essential for thriving in school and beyond. Here are strategies for integrating mindfulness into learning environments:

1. Mindful Breathing Exercises:
 - Start classes or lessons with brief mindful breathing exercises to help students transition into a focused and present state.
 - Teach students simple breathing techniques such as deep belly breathing, square breathing, or mindful counting to promote relaxation and concentration.

2. Mindful Movement Activities:
 - Incorporate mindful movement activities such as yoga, stretching, or tai chi into the daily routine to promote physical well-being and mindfulness.
 - Lead students through guided movement sequences that encourage mindful awareness of body sensations, breath, and movement.

3. Mindful Listening and Observation:
 - Encourage mindful listening and observation exercises to enhance attention, perception, and sensory awareness.
 - Engage students in activities such as mindful listening to sounds in the environment, observing nature mindfully, or mindful eating exercises.

4. Mindful Reflection and Journaling:
 - Integrate opportunities for mindful reflection and journaling into the curriculum to promote self-awareness, self-expression, and metacognition.

- Provide prompts for reflective writing, gratitude journaling, or mindful storytelling to help students process their thoughts, emotions, and experiences.

5. Mindful Communication and Empathy:

- Foster mindful communication skills and empathy through group discussions, role-playing activities, and cooperative learning experiences.
- Teach students active listening, compassionate speaking, and perspective-taking skills to enhance interpersonal relationships and conflict resolution.

6. Mindful Technology Use:

- Promote mindful technology use by encouraging students to engage with digital devices and screens mindfully.
- Teach digital mindfulness practices such as digital detoxes, mindful scrolling, or setting mindful intentions before using technology.

7. Mindful Classroom Management:

- Incorporate mindful classroom management strategies to create a calm and supportive learning environment.
- Use mindfulness-based techniques such as mindful transitions, mindful pauses, or mindful timeouts to manage behavior and promote emotional regulation.

8. Mindful Learning Activities:

- Design mindful learning activities that engage students in experiential, inquiry-based, and hands-on learning experiences.
- Integrate mindfulness into academic subjects through activities such as mindful reading, mindful math, or mindful science experiments.

9. Mindful Assessment and Feedback:

- Incorporate mindfulness into assessment and feedback practices to promote reflection, growth, and self-evaluation.
- Provide opportunities for students to reflect mindfully on their learning progress, set goals, and receive constructive feedback with openness and curiosity.

10. Cultivating a Mindful School Culture:
   - Foster a mindful school culture by modeling mindfulness practices, promoting staff well-being, and integrating mindfulness into school policies and practices.
   - Offer mindfulness training for educators, administrators, and staff to cultivate a shared language and understanding of mindfulness in the school community.

Nurturing Creativity and Emotional Intelligence

Nurturing creativity and emotional intelligence in educational settings is crucial for holistic development, as they play essential roles in shaping individuals' overall well-being, resilience, and success in life. Here's how educators can foster creativity and emotional intelligence in learning environments:

Nurturing Creativity:

1. Encourage Exploration and Curiosity:
   - Create a safe and supportive environment where students feel encouraged to explore new ideas, take risks, and think outside the box.
   - Provide open-ended learning experiences that allow for creative expression and experimentation across various subjects and disciplines.

2. Promote Playfulness and Imagination:
   - Incorporate playful activities, games, and imaginative storytelling into lessons to spark students' creativity and imagination.
   - Offer opportunities for dramatic play, role-playing, and improvisation to unleash students' creative potential and self-expression.

3. Value Divergent Thinking:
   - Emphasize divergent thinking skills by encouraging students to generate multiple solutions, perspectives, and interpretations to problems and challenges.
   - Provide prompts for brainstorming sessions, idea generation exercises, and creative problem-solving activities that foster divergent thinking skills.

4. Integrate Arts and Creative Practices:

- Integrate arts-based learning experiences such as visual arts, music, dance, theater, and creative writing into the curriculum to nurture students' creative expression and aesthetic appreciation.
- Offer opportunities for hands-on art projects, collaborative performances, and creative writing workshops that allow students to explore their interests and talents.

5. Support Risk-Taking and Failure:

- Create a culture that celebrates risk-taking, resilience, and learning from failure as essential components of the creative process.
- Encourage students to embrace setbacks, iterate on their ideas, and persevere through challenges, fostering a growth mindset and resilience in the face of adversity.

Fostering Emotional Intelligence:

1. Teach Self-Awareness:

- Help students develop self-awareness by encouraging reflection, mindfulness practices, and journaling to understand their thoughts, emotions, and behaviors.
- Provide opportunities for students to explore their strengths, values, and personal identities, fostering a deeper understanding of themselves.

2. Cultivate Empathy and Compassion:

- Foster empathy and compassion by promoting perspective-taking, active listening, and understanding of others' emotions and experiences.
- Incorporate cooperative learning activities, community service projects, and discussions about social justice issues to cultivate empathy and a sense of social responsibility.

3. Practice Emotion Regulation:

- Teach students effective emotion regulation strategies such as deep breathing, mindfulness, and positive self-talk to manage stress, anxiety, and strong emotions.

- Model healthy coping mechanisms and provide guidance on how to recognize and express emotions in constructive ways.

4. Build Healthy Relationships:
   - Provide opportunities for students to develop positive interpersonal skills and build healthy relationships with peers, teachers, and family members.
   - Teach communication skills, conflict resolution techniques, and assertiveness strategies to navigate social interactions and build meaningful connections.

5. Promote Emotional Expression:
   - Create a supportive environment where students feel comfortable expressing their emotions through art, writing, music, or verbal communication.
   - Encourage open dialogue about emotions, feelings, and mental health to reduce stigma and promote emotional well-being.

Holistic Approaches to Lifelong Learning

Holistic approaches to lifelong learning emphasize the continuous development of the whole person—physically, mentally, emotionally, socially, and spiritually—throughout one's lifetime. These approaches recognize that learning extends beyond formal education and encompasses various dimensions of human experience. Here are key principles and strategies for fostering holistic lifelong learning:

1. Cultivating Curiosity and Openness:
   - Encourage individuals to maintain a curious and open mindset, embracing learning opportunities in diverse areas of interest.
   - Promote a growth mindset that views challenges as opportunities for growth and learning rather than setbacks.

2. Integrating Mindfulness and Self-Reflection:
   - Incorporate mindfulness practices and self-reflection into daily routines to enhance self-awareness, clarity of thought, and emotional resilience.

- Encourage individuals to pause, reflect on their experiences, and extract valuable insights for personal growth and development.

3. Embracing Experiential Learning:
- Emphasize experiential learning opportunities that engage individuals in hands-on, real-world experiences, fostering deep understanding and practical skills.
- Encourage participation in internships, apprenticeships, volunteering, travel, and other experiential learning activities that promote holistic development.

4. Promoting Lifelong Health and Well-Being:
- Advocate for the integration of health and well-being practices into lifelong learning, including physical exercise, healthy nutrition, stress management, and mindfulness.
- Empower individuals to take proactive steps to maintain their physical, mental, and emotional well-being throughout their lives.

5. Fostering Personal Growth and Self-Actualization:
- Support individuals in pursuing personal growth and self-actualization by setting meaningful goals, exploring passions, and expanding their horizons.
- Encourage self-directed learning initiatives such as reading, attending workshops, pursuing hobbies, and engaging in creative endeavors.

6. Nurturing Emotional Intelligence and Interpersonal Skills:
- Foster the development of emotional intelligence and interpersonal skills, including empathy, communication, conflict resolution, and collaboration.
- Provide opportunities for individuals to cultivate healthy relationships, navigate social dynamics, and contribute positively to their communities.

7. Emphasizing Lifelong Learning Communities:
- Create and participate in lifelong learning communities that provide opportunities for collaboration, mentorship, and knowledge sharing.

- Facilitate peer-to-peer learning networks, study groups, book clubs, and online forums where individuals can connect, learn from each other, and support mutual growth.

8. Embracing Cultural and Global Awareness:

- Encourage individuals to embrace cultural diversity, develop intercultural competence, and engage with global issues and perspectives.
- Promote lifelong learning experiences that foster cross-cultural understanding, empathy, and appreciation for the richness of human diversity.

9. Supporting Continued Professional Development:

- Advocate for ongoing professional development and skill enhancement to adapt to changing career demands and technological advancements.
- Provide resources, training programs, and mentorship opportunities to support individuals in advancing their careers and achieving their professional goals.

10. Emphasizing Meaning and Purpose:

- Encourage individuals to seek learning experiences that align with their values, passions, and sense of purpose, fostering fulfillment and a sense of meaning in life.
- Support individuals in reflecting on their life goals, aspirations, and contributions to society, guiding them towards a holistic and purposeful life journey.

Building Holistic Educational Systems

Building holistic educational systems involves designing learning environments that prioritize the development of the whole person—physically, mentally, emotionally, socially, and spiritually. These systems aim to nurture the holistic well-being of students, educators, and communities, fostering a culture of learning excellence, equity, and empowerment. Here are key principles and strategies for building holistic educational systems:

1. Student-Centered Learning:
- Prioritize student agency, voice, and choice in the learning process, allowing students to pursue personalized learning pathways aligned with their interests, strengths, and aspirations.
- Create opportunities for student-led inquiry, project-based learning, and experiential learning experiences that promote active engagement and deep understanding.

2. Holistic Curriculum Design:
- Develop interdisciplinary and integrated curricula that address the diverse needs and interests of learners while fostering connections across subject areas and real-world contexts.
- Embed holistic education principles, including mindfulness, emotional intelligence, global citizenship, sustainability, and social justice, into the curriculum.

3. Culturally Responsive Practices:
- Embrace cultural diversity and promote inclusive practices that honor students' cultural backgrounds, languages, and identities.
- Incorporate culturally relevant content, perspectives, and teaching methodologies that reflect the diversity of students' experiences and contribute to their sense of belonging and cultural competence.

4. Supportive Learning Environments:
- Create safe, supportive, and nurturing learning environments that prioritize students' physical, emotional, and psychological well-being.
- Foster positive relationships, mutual respect, and a sense of community among students, educators, families, and other stakeholders.

5. Professional Development and Support:
- Provide ongoing professional development and support for educators to enhance their pedagogical skills, cultural competence, and well-being.
- Offer training in mindfulness, trauma-informed practices, restorative justice, social-emotional learning, and inclusive teaching strategies to equip educators with the tools they need to support holistic student development.

6. Social and Emotional Learning (SEL):
   - Integrate social and emotional learning (SEL) into the curriculum to promote students' self-awareness, self-management, social awareness, relationship skills, and responsible decision-making.
   - Implement evidence-based SEL programs and practices that address the holistic needs of students and contribute to positive academic, social, and emotional outcomes.

7. Family and Community Engagement:
   - Foster partnerships with families, communities, and external organizations to support holistic student development and well-being.
   - Engage families as partners in the educational process, involving them in decision-making, goal-setting, and collaborative initiatives that enhance student learning and success.

8. Technology Integration for Holistic Learning:
   - Leverage technology as a tool for holistic learning, creativity, and collaboration, while promoting responsible digital citizenship and well-being.
   - Integrate educational technologies that support personalized learning, inquiry-based exploration, and authentic connections with global communities.

9. Assessment for Learning and Growth:
   - Use a variety of assessment strategies, including formative assessment, performance-based assessment, portfolios, and self-assessment, to measure holistic student learning and growth.
   - Shift towards competency-based assessment models that focus on mastery of essential skills, knowledge, and dispositions aligned with holistic education goals.

10. Advocacy for Holistic Education:
   - Advocate for policies, funding, and resources that support holistic education approaches and address systemic barriers to equity and inclusion.
   - Collaborate with stakeholders at the local, regional, and national levels to promote holistic education principles and advance a shared vision of educational excellence and well-being for all.

Chapter 17
Holistic Perspectives on Weight Management

Mindful Eating for Weight Wellness

Mindful eating is a holistic approach to weight management that emphasizes awareness, presence, and intentionality in food consumption. It involves paying close attention to the sensory experiences, thoughts, and emotions associated with eating, without judgment or distraction. By practicing mindful eating, individuals can develop a healthier relationship with food, enhance their body awareness, and make more conscious choices that support their overall well-being. Here are key principles and strategies for incorporating mindful eating into weight wellness:

1. Cultivate Awareness:
  - **Mindful Presence:** Bring full awareness to the eating experience by slowing down, savoring each bite, and focusing on the present moment.
  - **Sensory Awareness:** Tune into the colors, textures, flavors, and aromas of food, engaging all the senses to fully experience the act of eating.
  - **Internal Cues:** Listen to the body's hunger and fullness signals, honoring its natural cues for nourishment and satisfaction.

2. Practice Non-Judgment:
  - **Release Judgment:** Let go of negative thoughts, guilt, or shame associated with food choices, and approach eating with a mindset of self-compassion and acceptance.
  - **Cultivate Curiosity:** Adopt a curious and open attitude towards food and eating experiences, exploring preferences, reactions, and patterns without criticism.

3. Honor Hunger and Fullness:
  - **Eat Mindfully:** Pay attention to physical hunger cues, such as stomach growling or low energy levels, before deciding to eat.
  - **Pause and Check-In:** Pause periodically during meals to assess hunger and fullness levels, aiming for a comfortable level of satisfaction without overeating or under-eating.

4. Engage Mindfully:

- **Eliminate Distractions:** Minimize distractions such as screens, work, or multitasking while eating, allowing for focused attention on the eating experience.
- **Slow Down:** Eat slowly and mindfully, chewing food thoroughly and taking breaks between bites to savor flavors and textures.

5. Cultivate Gratitude:

- **Gratitude Practice:** Cultivate gratitude for the nourishment provided by food, expressing appreciation for the effort and resources involved in its production.
- **Savor Moments:** Take moments to express gratitude before and after meals, acknowledging the interconnectedness of food, health, and well-being.

6. Tune into Emotional Eating:

- **Emotional Awareness:** Recognize the connection between emotions and eating behaviors, becoming aware of emotional triggers, cravings, and patterns.
- **Alternative Coping Strategies:** Develop alternative coping strategies for managing emotions, such as mindful breathing, journaling, or engaging in supportive activities.

7. Foster Mindful Food Choices:

- **Intuitive Eating:** Trust your body's wisdom to guide food choices based on hunger, cravings, and nutritional needs, rather than external rules or restrictions.
- **Nutritional Awareness:** Balance mindful eating with nutritional knowledge, aiming for a diverse and balanced diet that nourishes the body and supports overall health.

8. Practice Self-Compassion:

- **Self-Kindness:** Approach weight management with self-compassion and kindness, acknowledging that change takes time and effort, and embracing imperfection along the journey.
- **Gentle Awareness:** Notice and gently redirect unhelpful thoughts or behaviors related to weight management, replacing self-criticism with self-care and encouragement.

9. Reflect and Learn:

- **Reflective Practice:** Reflect on eating experiences without judgment, noticing how different foods, environments, and emotions impact your well-being.
- **Learn from Experience:** Use insights gained from mindful eating to make informed choices and adjustments that support your weight wellness goals over time.

10. Seek Support and Guidance:
- **Community Connection:** Seek support from like-minded individuals, friends, or family members who share your commitment to mindful eating and weight wellness.
- **Professional Guidance:** Consider working with a registered dietitian, therapist, or mindfulness coach who specializes in mindful eating and can provide personalized guidance and support.

Holistic Approaches to Exercise and Fitness

Holistic approaches to exercise and fitness focus on integrating physical activity into a balanced lifestyle that promotes overall well-being, rather than solely focusing on weight loss or aesthetic goals. These approaches prioritize movement that supports the mind, body, and spirit, emphasizing enjoyment, sustainability, and alignment with individual needs and preferences. Here are key principles and strategies for incorporating holistic approaches to exercise and fitness:

1. Mindful Movement:
- **Mind-Body Connection:** Choose activities that foster a strong mind-body connection, such as yoga, Pilates, tai chi, or qigong, which promote awareness, breath control, and mental relaxation.
- **Intention Setting:** Approach exercise with intention and mindfulness, focusing on how movement makes you feel rather than solely on calorie burning or performance metrics.

2. Variety and Adaptability:
- **Diverse Activities:** Engage in a variety of physical activities that provide different benefits and experiences, including cardiovascular exercise, strength training, flexibility work, and outdoor activities.

- **Adapt to Needs:** Listen to your body and adapt your exercise routine to accommodate changing needs, energy levels, and preferences over time.

3. Functional Fitness:
- **Functional Movement:** Incorporate exercises that mimic everyday movements and improve functional fitness, such as squatting, lifting, pushing, and pulling, to enhance mobility, stability, and overall physical function.
- **Balance and Coordination:** Include exercises that challenge balance, coordination, and proprioception, such as balance drills, agility exercises, and proprioceptive training, to improve overall movement quality.

4. Joyful Movement:
- **Find Enjoyment:** Choose activities that bring you joy and pleasure, whether it's dancing, hiking, cycling, gardening, or playing recreational sports, to make exercise a sustainable and fulfilling part of your lifestyle.
- **Playful Approach:** Embrace a playful and lighthearted attitude towards movement, exploring new activities and environments with curiosity and enthusiasm.

5. Holistic Health Focus:
- **Wellness Integration:** Integrate exercise into a holistic wellness routine that includes nutrition, sleep, stress management, and self-care practices, recognizing that physical activity is just one aspect of overall health.
- **Rest and Recovery:** Prioritize rest and recovery alongside physical activity, allowing time for relaxation, sleep, and rejuvenation to support optimal recovery and adaptation.

6. Connection and Community:
- **Social Engagement:** Participate in group fitness classes, team sports, or outdoor recreation activities to foster social connections, accountability, and a sense of community.
- **Supportive Environment:** Surround yourself with supportive and like-minded individuals who share your commitment to holistic health

and fitness goals, providing encouragement, motivation, and camaraderie.

7. Nature and Outdoor Exercise:
  - **Nature Connection:** Take advantage of opportunities to exercise outdoors in natural settings, such as parks, trails, beaches, or forests, to benefit from the restorative effects of nature on physical and mental well-being.
  - **Earthing Practices:** Practice earthing or grounding by walking barefoot on natural surfaces, such as grass or sand, to connect with the Earth's energy and enhance vitality and resilience.

8. Mindful Recovery:
  - **Active Recovery:** Incorporate active recovery techniques, such as gentle yoga, foam rolling, or mobility exercises, into your routine to promote circulation, reduce muscle tension, and support recovery after intense workouts.
  - **Mindfulness Practices:** Use mindfulness techniques, such as meditation, deep breathing, or progressive relaxation, to promote relaxation, reduce stress, and enhance recovery between exercise sessions.

9. Self-Compassion and Acceptance:
  - **Body Positivity:** Practice body positivity and self-acceptance, recognizing that all bodies are worthy of care and respect regardless of size, shape, or fitness level.
  - **Focus on Health:** Shift the focus from external appearance or weight-related goals to health-enhancing behaviors and markers, such as improved strength, stamina, flexibility, and energy levels.

10. Personalized Approach:
  - **Individualized Programming:** Tailor your exercise routine to suit your unique preferences, goals, and physical capabilities, seeking guidance from fitness professionals or health practitioners as needed.
  - **Listen to Your Body:** Honor your body's signals and limitations, adjusting your exercise intensity, duration, and frequency based on how you feel and what your body needs in the moment.

Emotional Well-Being and Weight Management

Emotional well-being plays a crucial role in weight management within a holistic health framework. Emotional eating, stress, self-esteem, and mental health all intertwine with dietary habits and physical activity levels. Here's how emotional well-being influences weight management and strategies to foster a healthy balance:

1. Understanding Emotional Eating:
 - **Emotional Triggers:** Recognize emotional triggers that lead to overeating or unhealthy eating habits, such as stress, boredom, loneliness, or sadness.
 - **Mindful Awareness:** Practice mindful eating to distinguish between physical hunger and emotional hunger, allowing for more conscious food choices and eating behaviors.

2. Stress Management:
 - **Stress Response:** Understand how stress affects appetite, food cravings, and metabolism, often leading to emotional eating and weight gain.
 - **Stress Reduction Techniques:** Incorporate stress reduction techniques into daily life, such as meditation, deep breathing exercises, yoga, or spending time in nature, to mitigate the impact of stress on eating habits and weight management.

3. Positive Self-Image and Self-Esteem:
 - **Body Positivity:** Cultivate a positive body image and self-esteem, focusing on self-acceptance, self-compassion, and appreciation for body diversity.
 - **Healthy Mindset:** Shift the focus from weight loss to overall health and well-being, valuing internal qualities and achievements beyond external appearance.

4. Addressing Underlying Emotional Issues:
 - **Therapeutic Support:** Seek professional support from therapists, counselors, or support groups to address underlying emotional issues, trauma, or negative beliefs that contribute to disordered eating patterns or weight struggles.

  - **Cognitive-Behavioral Strategies:** Learn cognitive-behavioral strategies to challenge negative thought patterns, develop coping skills, and build resilience in managing emotions without turning to food for comfort.

5. Mind-Body Practices:
  - **Mindfulness and Meditation:** Practice mindfulness and meditation techniques to cultivate present-moment awareness, emotional regulation, and self-compassion, reducing the urge to use food as a coping mechanism.
  - **Yoga and Tai Chi:** Engage in mind-body practices such as yoga, tai chi, or qigong, which promote relaxation, stress reduction, and body awareness, fostering a positive relationship with both body and mind.

6. Social Support and Connection:
  - **Supportive Relationships:** Surround yourself with supportive friends, family members, or support groups who encourage positive health behaviors and provide emotional support during challenging times.
  - **Open Communication:** Communicate openly with loved ones about your emotional struggles or challenges with weight management, seeking understanding and encouragement without judgment.

7. Holistic Self-Care:
  - **Holistic Wellness Practices:** Prioritize holistic self-care practices that nurture emotional well-being, such as adequate sleep, regular physical activity, creative expression, time in nature, and meaningful social connections.
  - **Self-Compassionate Approach:** Adopt a self-compassionate approach to self-care, recognizing the importance of rest, relaxation, and self-nurturing activities in maintaining emotional balance and resilience.

8. Balanced Lifestyle:
  - **Healthy Coping Mechanisms:** Develop alternative coping mechanisms and stress management strategies that promote emotional well-being without relying on food, such as journaling, art therapy, or engaging in hobbies and interests.

- **Work-Life Balance:** Strive for a balanced lifestyle that includes time for relaxation, leisure activities, and self-care alongside work and other responsibilities, fostering a sense of fulfillment and satisfaction beyond food.

9. Professional Guidance:

- **Nutritional Counseling:** Seek guidance from registered dietitians or nutrition professionals who can provide personalized recommendations for managing emotional eating, improving dietary habits, and achieving weight-related goals.
- **Therapeutic Interventions:** Consider therapeutic interventions such as cognitive-behavioral therapy (CBT), dialectical behavior therapy (DBT), or acceptance and commitment therapy (ACT) to address emotional challenges and support weight management efforts.

10. Embracing Imperfection and Resilience:

- **Resilient Mindset:** Embrace imperfection and setbacks as part of the journey toward emotional well-being and weight management, cultivating resilience and perseverance in facing challenges.
- **Celebrate Progress:** Celebrate small victories and progress in developing healthier habits and coping mechanisms, acknowledging the importance of self-care and self-compassion along the way.

Addressing Underlying Health Factors in Weight

Addressing underlying health factors is essential in holistic weight management as it allows individuals to understand and address the root causes of weight-related issues rather than solely focusing on superficial solutions. Here's how to approach underlying health factors in weight management holistically:

1. Medical Evaluation:

- **Comprehensive Assessment:** Seek a thorough medical evaluation from healthcare professionals to identify underlying health conditions or factors contributing to weight-related issues.
- **Diagnostic Testing:** Undergo appropriate diagnostic tests, such as blood tests, hormonal assessments, thyroid function tests, or metabolic

evaluations, to identify any medical conditions affecting metabolism, hormones, or nutrient absorption.

2. Nutritional Considerations:
- **Nutrient Deficiencies:** Address nutritional deficiencies or imbalances that may impact weight management, such as deficiencies in vitamins, minerals, or essential nutrients required for metabolic health.
- **Nutritional Counseling:** Consult with a registered dietitian or nutritionist to develop a personalized nutrition plan that addresses individual dietary needs, preferences, and health goals, emphasizing whole foods, balanced macronutrients, and nutrient-dense choices.

3. Hormonal Imbalances:
- **Hormonal Evaluation:** Evaluate hormonal imbalances, such as insulin resistance, thyroid dysfunction, cortisol dysregulation, or reproductive hormone imbalances, which can affect metabolism, appetite regulation, and weight distribution.
- **Hormone Regulation:** Work with healthcare providers to regulate hormone levels through lifestyle modifications, medication management, or hormone replacement therapy as appropriate, addressing underlying imbalances contributing to weight issues.

4. Gut Health Optimization:
- **Gut Microbiome Assessment:** Consider assessing gut health and microbiome composition to identify imbalances or dysbiosis that may impact digestion, nutrient absorption, inflammation, and metabolic health.
- **Gut Healing Protocols:** Implement gut-healing protocols, such as probiotic supplementation, prebiotic-rich foods, fermented foods, and dietary fiber, to support a healthy gut environment and optimize metabolic function.

5. Metabolic Health:
- **Metabolic Testing:** Assess metabolic health parameters, including metabolic rate, insulin sensitivity, lipid profile, and blood glucose levels, to identify metabolic dysregulation or abnormalities contributing to weight management challenges.

- **Metabolic Interventions:** Explore metabolic interventions such as dietary modifications, physical activity, intermittent fasting, or metabolic conditioning exercises to improve metabolic flexibility, insulin sensitivity, and metabolic health outcomes.

6. Sleep Quality and Patterns:

- **Sleep Evaluation:** Evaluate sleep quality, duration, and patterns to identify sleep-related issues such as sleep apnea, insomnia, or circadian rhythm disturbances that may impact metabolism, appetite regulation, and weight management.
- **Sleep Hygiene Practices:** Implement sleep hygiene practices to optimize sleep quality and duration, including maintaining a consistent sleep schedule, creating a conducive sleep environment, limiting screen time before bed, and practicing relaxation techniques.

7. Stress Management:

- **Stress Assessment:** Assess stress levels and identify sources of chronic stress, emotional tension, or psychological distress that may contribute to weight gain, emotional eating, or hormonal imbalances.
- **Stress Reduction Strategies:** Incorporate stress reduction strategies such as mindfulness meditation, deep breathing exercises, yoga, or relaxation techniques to mitigate the impact of stress on metabolism, appetite regulation, and weight management.

8. Medication Review:

- **Medication Evaluation:** Review current medications, including prescription drugs, over-the-counter medications, or supplements, to identify any medications that may affect weight or metabolism as a side effect.
- **Medication Adjustment:** Work with healthcare providers to adjust medication regimens as needed, exploring alternative medications with fewer metabolic side effects or exploring non-pharmacological interventions to manage health conditions.

9. Mental Health and Emotional Well-Being:

- **Psychological Assessment:** Evaluate mental health status, emotional well-being, and psychological factors contributing to weight management challenges, such as depression, anxiety, trauma, or disordered eating behaviors.

- **Psychotherapeutic Interventions:** Engage in psychotherapeutic interventions such as cognitive-behavioral therapy (CBT), dialectical behavior therapy (DBT), or acceptance and commitment therapy (ACT) to address underlying emotional issues, develop coping skills, and support holistic weight management.

10. **Holistic Approach Integration:**
 - **Multidisciplinary Collaboration:** Foster collaboration among healthcare providers, including physicians, dietitians, therapists, and other allied health professionals, to address underlying health factors in a comprehensive and integrated manner.
 - **Holistic Lifestyle Modification:** Embrace holistic lifestyle modifications that address physical, emotional, mental, and spiritual aspects of health, fostering a balanced approach to weight management that prioritizes overall well-being and vitality.

Holistic Perspectives on Body Image

Holistic perspectives on body image emphasize cultivating a positive relationship with one's body that goes beyond physical appearance and embraces overall well-being, self-acceptance, and self-compassion. Here are key aspects of holistic body image perspectives:

1. **Self-Acceptance and Self-Compassion:**
 - **Unconditional Self-Worth:** Foster a sense of unconditional self-worth and self-acceptance, recognizing that self-worth is not contingent on external appearance or adherence to societal beauty standards.
 - **Self-Compassionate Mindset:** Cultivate self-compassion by treating oneself with kindness, understanding, and non-judgment, particularly during times of body dissatisfaction or perceived flaws.

2. **Embracing Body Diversity:**
 - **Body Neutrality:** Shift focus from body positivity to body neutrality, acknowledging that all bodies are inherently valuable and worthy of respect regardless of size, shape, or appearance.

- **Celebrating Diversity:** Celebrate the diversity of body shapes, sizes, abilities, and identities, recognizing the beauty and uniqueness of each individual's body.

3. Mindful Body Awareness:

- **Embodied Mindfulness:** Practice embodied mindfulness by tuning into bodily sensations, emotions, and needs without judgment, fostering a deeper connection with one's body and promoting self-awareness.
- **Intuitive Body Wisdom:** Listen to the body's cues for hunger, fullness, and satisfaction, honoring its natural signals and promoting a balanced approach to eating and movement.

4. Holistic Health Focus:

- **Health at Every Size (HAES):** Embrace the Health at Every Size (HAES) paradigm, which promotes health-focused behaviors rather than weight-centered goals, emphasizing holistic health markers such as physical fitness, mental well-being, and overall vitality.
- **Wellness-Centered Goals:** Set wellness-centered goals that prioritize behaviors supporting physical, emotional, and mental well-being, rather than solely focusing on weight loss or achieving a certain body size.

5. Media Literacy and Critical Thinking:

- **Media Awareness:** Develop media literacy skills to critically evaluate and challenge unrealistic beauty ideals portrayed in mainstream media, recognizing the role of media in shaping societal beauty standards and body image perceptions.
- **Body-Positive Media Representation:** Seek out diverse and inclusive media representations that reflect a wide range of body types, promoting body positivity and challenging narrow beauty standards.

6. Holistic Self-Care Practices:

- **Self-Nurturing Activities:** Engage in self-care practices that nurture overall well-being, including adequate sleep, stress management, physical activity, creative expression, and meaningful social connections.

- **Self-Expression:** Express yourself authentically through fashion, art, movement, or other forms of self-expression, embracing individuality and celebrating your unique identity.

7. Healthy Relationships and Support:
- **Supportive Environment:** Surround yourself with supportive friends, family members, or communities who value you for who you are beyond your physical appearance, fostering a sense of belonging and acceptance.
- **Open Communication:** Communicate openly with loved ones about body image struggles, seeking understanding, empathy, and encouragement without judgment or criticism.

8. Body-Positive Movement:
- **Body-Inclusive Activism:** Participate in body-positive activism and advocacy efforts that challenge weight stigma, promote body diversity, and advocate for social justice and inclusivity in healthcare, media, and society.
- **Community Engagement:** Engage in body-positive communities and movements that empower individuals to embrace their bodies, challenge oppressive beauty standards, and support each other in their journey towards self-love and acceptance.

9. Professional Support and Healing:
- **Therapeutic Interventions:** Seek support from therapists, counselors, or body image specialists who can provide therapeutic interventions such as cognitive-behavioral therapy (CBT), body image-focused therapy, or acceptance and commitment therapy (ACT) to address body image concerns and foster self-acceptance.
- **Healing Trauma:** Address underlying trauma or experiences of body shaming, discrimination, or abuse that may contribute to negative body image, seeking healing and support through trauma-informed therapies and interventions.

10. Holistic Mind-Body-Spirit Integration:
- **Spiritual Connection:** Cultivate a spiritual connection or sense of purpose that transcends physical appearance, tapping into inner resources of strength, resilience, and wisdom to navigate challenges and cultivate holistic well-being.

- **Wholeness and Integration:** Embrace a holistic perspective of health that integrates mind, body, and spirit, recognizing that true well-being comes from nurturing all aspects of oneself and finding harmony within.

205

Chapter 18
Holistic Practices for Stress Management

Mind-Body Techniques for Stress Reduction

Incorporating mind-body techniques into your routine can be incredibly effective for managing stress holistically. These practices not only help to alleviate the physical symptoms of stress but also promote relaxation, emotional balance, and overall well-being. Here are some powerful mind-body techniques for stress reduction:

1. Mindfulness Meditation:
   - **Practice:** Set aside time each day for mindfulness meditation. Sit comfortably, focus on your breath or a mantra, and gently redirect your attention back whenever your mind wanders.
   - **Benefits:** Mindfulness meditation helps cultivate present-moment awareness, reduces rumination, and enhances resilience to stressors.

2. Deep Breathing Exercises (Pranayama):
   - **Techniques:** Try diaphragmatic breathing, box breathing, or alternate nostril breathing. Inhale deeply through your nose, fill your lungs, hold briefly, and exhale slowly through your mouth.
   - **Benefits:** Deep breathing triggers the relaxation response, lowers heart rate and blood pressure, and promotes a state of calmness and relaxation.

3. Progressive Muscle Relaxation (PMR):
   - **Practice:** Starting from your toes, tense and then relax each muscle group in your body sequentially, working your way up to your head. Hold tension for a few seconds before releasing.
   - **Benefits:** PMR reduces muscle tension, relieves physical symptoms of stress, and promotes relaxation and body awareness.

4. Yoga and Tai Chi:
   - **Practices:** Engage in yoga poses (asanas) or tai chi movements that focus on breath awareness, gentle stretching, and mindful movement.
   - **Benefits:** Yoga and tai chi improve flexibility, balance, and strength, while also calming the mind, reducing stress hormones, and promoting relaxation.

5. Guided Imagery and Visualization:

- **Process:** Close your eyes and imagine yourself in a peaceful, serene environment. Use all your senses to vividly imagine the sights, sounds, smells, and sensations of this place.
- **Benefits:** Guided imagery induces relaxation, reduces anxiety, and helps shift focus away from stressors to positive mental images.

6. Body Scan Meditation:
- **Practice:** Lie down or sit comfortably and systematically scan your body from head to toe, observing any tension, discomfort, or sensations without judgment.
- **Benefits:** Body scan meditation promotes relaxation, body awareness, and mindfulness, helping to release physical tension and reduce stress.

7. Biofeedback Therapy:
- **Process:** Use biofeedback devices to monitor physiological responses such as heart rate variability, muscle tension, or skin conductance, and learn to regulate these responses through relaxation techniques.
- **Benefits:** Biofeedback enhances self-awareness, teaches self-regulation skills, and promotes relaxation and stress reduction.

8. Autogenic Training:
- **Technique:** Practice self-generated relaxation through repeated affirmations focused on warmth, heaviness, and relaxation in different parts of the body.
- **Benefits:** Autogenic training induces deep relaxation, reduces muscle tension, and calms the autonomic nervous system.

9. Mindful Walking:
- **Practice:** Take a slow, mindful walk outdoors, paying attention to each step, the sensations of walking, and the surrounding environment.
- **Benefits:** Mindful walking promotes grounding, stress reduction, and connection with nature, fostering a sense of calmness and presence.

10. Journaling and Expressive Writing:

- **Process:** Write about your thoughts, feelings, and experiences related to stressors, challenges, or emotions. Allow yourself to express freely without judgment.
- **Benefits:** Journaling promotes emotional processing, self-reflection, and stress release, providing clarity and insight into stress triggers and coping strategies.

Integrating Relaxation Practices into Daily Life

Integrating relaxation practices into your daily life is essential for managing stress and promoting overall well-being. By incorporating these practices into your routine, you can create moments of calm and rejuvenation amidst the demands of daily life. Here are some effective ways to integrate relaxation practices into your daily routine:

1. Morning Rituals:
- **Mindful Wake-Up:** Start your day with a few minutes of deep breathing or gentle stretching to awaken your body and mind mindfully.
- **Gratitude Practice:** Begin each day by expressing gratitude for the blessings in your life, fostering a positive mindset and setting the tone for the day ahead.

2. Mindful Moments Throughout the Day:
- **Breath Breaks:** Take short breaks throughout the day to practice deep breathing exercises, bringing your focus back to the present moment and relieving tension.
- **Mindful Eating:** Practice mindful eating by savoring each bite, paying attention to flavors, textures, and sensations, and cultivating awareness of hunger and fullness cues.

3. Nature Breaks:
- **Outdoor Walks:** Take short walks in nature during breaks or lunchtime, connecting with the natural world, and refreshing your mind and body.
- **Gardening or Outdoor Activities:** Engage in gardening, outdoor yoga, or other activities that allow you to connect with nature and reap the benefits of sunlight and fresh air.

4. Midday Relaxation:
  - **Mini Meditation:** Dedicate a few minutes to meditation or visualization during your lunch break, calming your mind and resetting for the rest of the day.
  - **Progressive Muscle Relaxation:** Practice progressive muscle relaxation at your desk or in a quiet space to release tension and promote relaxation.

5. Afternoon Recharge:
  - **Power Nap:** Take a short power nap during the afternoon to recharge your energy levels and boost mental clarity and productivity.
  - **Deep Breathing Breaks:** Schedule regular deep breathing breaks to prevent mid-afternoon slumps and maintain focus and vitality.

6. Evening Wind-Down:
  - **Mindful Movement:** Practice gentle yoga or tai chi in the evening to unwind from the day's stressors and prepare your body for restful sleep.
  - **Warm Bath:** Take a warm bath infused with essential oils like lavender or chamomile to relax your muscles and soothe your mind before bedtime.

7. Digital Detox:
  - **Screen-Free Time:** Allocate dedicated periods of time each day to disconnect from electronic devices and engage in activities that promote relaxation and connection with loved ones.
  - **Quiet Evening Rituals:** Create a technology-free zone in the evening to promote relaxation and prepare your mind for restful sleep.

8. Bedtime Rituals:
  - **Relaxing Rituals:** Establish bedtime rituals such as reading, journaling, or practicing relaxation exercises to signal to your body that it's time to wind down.
  - **Mindful Reflection:** Reflect on your day with kindness and compassion, letting go of any stress or worries before drifting off to sleep.

9. Breath Awareness Throughout the Day:

- **Anchor Breathing:** Use your breath as an anchor throughout the day, returning to your breath whenever you feel overwhelmed or stressed, and using it as a tool to ground yourself in the present moment.
- **Breath Reminders:** Set reminders on your phone or computer to take mindful breathing breaks at regular intervals, helping you maintain a sense of calm and balance amidst daily challenges.

10. Gratitude Practice Before Bed:
- **Gratitude Journaling:** End your day by writing down three things you're grateful for, cultivating a sense of appreciation and contentment as you prepare for sleep.
- **Loving-Kindness Meditation:** Practice a loving-kindness meditation before bed, sending wishes of well-being and happiness to yourself and others, fostering a sense of connection and compassion.

Holistic Approaches to Work-Related Stress

Holistic approaches to work-related stress involve addressing the root causes of stress while implementing strategies that promote overall well-being in the workplace. Here are some holistic practices for managing work-related stress:

1. Work-Life Balance:
- **Setting Boundaries:** Establish clear boundaries between work and personal life, including designated work hours and dedicated time for relaxation, hobbies, and social activities.
- **Prioritizing Self-Care:** Prioritize self-care activities such as exercise, meditation, and spending time with loved ones, recognizing that your well-being is essential for productivity and resilience.

2. Mindful Work Practices:
- **Mindful Time Management:** Practice mindful time management techniques or time-blocking to increase focus, productivity, and efficiency while reducing stress.
- **Single-Tasking:** Focus on one task at a time, avoiding multitasking, which can increase stress and decrease the quality of work.

3. Stress-Reduction Techniques:
   - **Breathing Exercises:** Incorporate deep breathing exercises or mindfulness meditation breaks throughout the workday to reduce stress, increase focus, and promote relaxation.
   - **Progressive Muscle Relaxation:** Practice progressive muscle relaxation at your desk or during breaks to release tension and promote physical and mental relaxation.

4. Physical Movement and Ergonomics:
   - **Regular Movement Breaks:** Take short movement breaks every hour to stretch, walk around, or do simple exercises to relieve physical tension and improve circulation.
   - **Ergonomic Workspace:** Ensure your workspace is ergonomically designed to minimize physical strain and discomfort, including proper desk setup, chair height, and monitor placement.

5. Healthy Nutrition and Hydration:
   - **Balanced Meals:** Fuel your body with nutritious, balanced meals and snacks throughout the workday to support energy levels, mood stability, and cognitive function.
   - **Hydration:** Stay hydrated by drinking plenty of water throughout the day, as dehydration can exacerbate stress and fatigue.

6. Social Support and Connection:
   - **Building Relationships:** Cultivate supportive relationships with colleagues and supervisors, fostering a sense of camaraderie, teamwork, and emotional support in the workplace.
   - **Seeking Support:** Reach out to trusted coworkers, mentors, or Employee Assistance Programs (EAPs) for guidance, advice, and assistance in managing work-related stressors.

7. Time Management and Organization:
   - **Prioritizing Tasks:** Use task prioritization techniques such as the Eisenhower Matrix or ABC method to identify and focus on high-priority tasks, reducing overwhelm and increasing productivity.
   - **Effective Delegation:** Delegate tasks when possible, recognizing your limits and empowering team members to contribute their skills and expertise.

8. Mindful Communication:
- **Clear Communication:** Practice clear and assertive communication with coworkers and supervisors, expressing needs, boundaries, and concerns in a respectful and constructive manner.
- **Active Listening:** Practice active listening skills, empathetically tuning in to others' perspectives and concerns, fostering understanding and collaboration in the workplace.

9. Professional Development and Growth:
- **Learning Opportunities:** Seek out opportunities for professional development and skill enhancement to build confidence, competence, and resilience in handling work-related challenges.
- **Work-Life Integration:** Find ways to integrate personal interests, passions, and values into your work, promoting a sense of purpose, fulfillment, and alignment with your holistic well-being.

10. Self-Reflection and Adaptation:
- **Regular Check-Ins:** Take time to reflect on your work habits, stress triggers, and coping strategies, adjusting your approach as needed to better manage stress and promote well-being.
- **Flexibility and Adaptability:** Cultivate a flexible mindset and adaptability to navigate change, uncertainty, and unexpected challenges in the workplace with resilience and grace.

Mindful Approaches to Financial Stress

Mindful approaches to financial stress involve cultivating awareness and adopting intentional strategies to manage and alleviate the emotional and psychological burdens associated with financial challenges. Here are some holistic practices for managing financial stress mindfully:

1. Mindful Budgeting:
- **Awareness of Spending Habits:** Practice mindful awareness of your spending habits, tracking expenses, and identifying areas where you can reduce discretionary spending.
- **Values-Based Budgeting:** Align your financial goals and priorities with your core values, allocating resources intentionally to support what matters most to you.

2. Practicing Gratitude:

- **Focus on Abundance:** Cultivate gratitude for what you have rather than dwelling on scarcity or financial struggles. Reflect on the positive aspects of your life and the non-material sources of happiness and fulfillment.
- **Gratitude Journaling:** Keep a gratitude journal to regularly write down things you're thankful for, fostering a positive mindset and resilience in the face of financial challenges.

3. Mindful Spending Decisions:

- **Conscious Consumption:** Practice mindful spending by pausing before making purchases and considering whether they align with your values and long-term financial goals.
- **Differentiating Needs and Wants:** Differentiate between essential needs and discretionary wants, prioritizing spending on necessities while minimizing non-essential expenses.

4. Stress Reduction Practices:

- **Mindfulness Meditation:** Engage in mindfulness meditation to cultivate present-moment awareness and reduce anxiety and stress related to financial concerns.
- **Deep Breathing Exercises:** Practice deep breathing exercises to calm the nervous system and promote relaxation during times of financial worry.

5. Creating Financial Plans:

- **Setting Realistic Goals:** Establish realistic and achievable financial goals, breaking them down into actionable steps to create a sense of progress and empowerment.
- **Emergency Fund:** Build an emergency fund to provide a financial safety net and reduce anxiety about unexpected expenses or emergencies.

6. Seeking Support:

- **Open Communication:** Foster open and honest communication with loved ones about financial concerns, seeking support and collaboration in finding solutions together.

- **Financial Counseling:** Consider seeking guidance from financial advisors or counselors who can provide objective advice and assistance in developing effective financial strategies.

7. Self-Compassion and Acceptance:
- **Cultivating Compassion:** Practice self-compassion and self-acceptance, recognizing that financial challenges are a normal part of life and refraining from self-criticism or judgment.
- **Letting Go of Perfectionism:** Release unrealistic expectations and perfectionist tendencies related to financial success, embracing imperfection and learning from setbacks with self-compassion.

8. Mindful Work and Career Choices:
- **Aligning Work with Values:** Consider whether your work aligns with your values and long-term goals, exploring opportunities for career growth and fulfillment that contribute to financial stability and well-being.
- **Work-Life Balance:** Prioritize work-life balance and self-care to prevent burnout and maintain resilience in navigating financial challenges.

9. Financial Education and Empowerment:
- **Continuous Learning:** Invest in financial education and literacy to build confidence and competence in managing finances effectively, empowering yourself to make informed decisions.
- **Seeking Resources:** Explore resources such as books, workshops, or online courses on personal finance to expand your knowledge and skills in managing money mindfully.

10. Living Within Means:
- **Sustainable Lifestyle:** Embrace a lifestyle that aligns with your financial means, focusing on sustainable and mindful consumption habits that support long-term financial well-being.
- **Gratitude for Simplicity:** Cultivate gratitude for simple pleasures and experiences that don't require significant financial resources, finding joy and contentment in the present moment.

Building Resilience Through Holistic Stress Management

Building resilience through holistic stress management involves adopting a comprehensive approach that addresses the mind, body, and spirit. By integrating various practices and strategies, you can strengthen your ability to cope with stressors and bounce back from adversity. Here are holistic practices for building resilience:

1. Mindfulness Meditation:
- **Mindful Awareness:** Practice mindfulness meditation to cultivate present-moment awareness and non-judgmental acceptance of your thoughts, emotions, and sensations.
- **Stress Reduction:** Use mindfulness techniques to observe and acknowledge stressors without becoming overwhelmed by them, promoting a sense of calm and perspective.

2. Physical Activity:
- **Regular Exercise:** Engage in regular physical activity such as walking, jogging, yoga, or swimming to reduce stress hormones, boost mood-enhancing neurotransmitters, and enhance overall resilience.
- **Mindful Movement:** Practice mindful movement activities like tai chi or qigong, which combine gentle physical exercise with breath awareness and meditation to promote relaxation and resilience.

3. Healthy Lifestyle Habits:
- **Balanced Nutrition:** Maintain a balanced diet rich in whole foods, fruits, vegetables, and lean proteins to support physical health and resilience against stress.
- **Adequate Sleep:** Prioritize restful sleep by establishing a consistent sleep schedule, creating a relaxing bedtime routine, and creating a comfortable sleep environment to enhance resilience and well-being.

4. Stress Reduction Techniques:
- **Breathing Exercises:** Practice deep breathing exercises, such as diaphragmatic breathing or box breathing, to activate the body's relaxation response and reduce stress levels.

- **Progressive Muscle Relaxation:** Incorporate progressive muscle relaxation techniques to release tension and promote physical and mental relaxation, fostering resilience against stress.

5. Social Support:
- **Building Relationships:** Cultivate supportive relationships with friends, family, or community members who offer emotional support, encouragement, and a sense of belonging during challenging times.
- **Connection:** Stay connected with loved ones through regular communication, shared activities, and expressions of care and empathy, enhancing resilience through social support.

6. Emotional Well-Being Practices:
- **Self-Compassion:** Cultivate self-compassion by treating yourself with kindness, understanding, and acceptance during times of stress or difficulty, fostering resilience in the face of adversity.
- **Positive Affirmations:** Practice positive self-talk and affirmations to challenge negative thoughts and beliefs, promoting resilience and a sense of self-efficacy.

7. Mind-Body Therapies:
- **Yoga and Meditation:** Incorporate yoga and meditation practices into your routine to promote relaxation, stress reduction, and emotional balance, enhancing resilience and coping skills.
- **Acupuncture or Massage:** Explore mind-body therapies such as acupuncture or massage therapy to alleviate physical tension, promote relaxation, and enhance overall resilience against stress.

8. Cognitive Strategies:
- **Cognitive Restructuring:** Challenge negative thought patterns and cognitive distortions through cognitive restructuring techniques, promoting resilience and adaptive coping strategies.
- **Problem-Solving Skills:** Develop problem-solving skills to effectively identify and address stressors, fostering resilience and proactive coping strategies.

9. Spiritual Practices:

- **Spiritual Connection:** Cultivate a sense of spirituality or connection to something greater than yourself through practices such as prayer, meditation, or reflection, fostering resilience and inner strength.
- **Purpose and Meaning:** Reflect on your values, purpose, and sense of meaning in life, drawing upon spiritual beliefs or principles to navigate challenges with resilience and perspective.

10. Holistic Self-Care:

- **Self-Care Rituals:** Establish regular self-care rituals that nurture your mind, body, and spirit, such as taking relaxing baths, enjoying nature walks, or engaging in creative hobbies, promoting resilience and well-being.

Chapter 19
Holistic Travel and Well-Being

Maintaining Holistic Practices While Traveling

Maintaining holistic practices while traveling is essential for preserving your overall well-being and ensuring a fulfilling travel experience. Here are some tips for incorporating holistic health practices into your travels:

1. Mindful Eating:
   - **Healthy Food Choices:** Prioritize nutritious, whole foods whenever possible, opting for fruits, vegetables, lean proteins, and whole grains to fuel your body and support energy levels.
   - **Local Cuisine:** Explore local cuisine that reflects the culture and flavors of your destination while making mindful choices that align with your dietary preferences and health goals.

2. Physical Activity:
   - **Stay Active:** Incorporate physical activity into your travel itinerary by exploring on foot, renting bikes, or participating in outdoor activities like hiking, swimming, or yoga.
   - **Hotel Workouts:** Utilize hotel gyms or fitness centers for workouts, or engage in bodyweight exercises and stretching routines in your hotel room to maintain fitness while traveling.

3. Stress Management:
   - **Mindfulness Practices:** Dedicate time for mindfulness meditation, deep breathing exercises, or mindful walks to reduce stress, enhance relaxation, and promote mental clarity during your travels.
   - **Unplug and Disconnect:** Take breaks from technology and immerse yourself in the present moment, enjoying the sights, sounds, and experiences of your destination without distractions.

4. Sleep Hygiene:
   - **Consistent Sleep Routine:** Maintain a consistent sleep schedule, even while traveling, by prioritizing restful sleep and creating a comfortable sleep environment conducive to relaxation and rejuvenation.
   - **Jet Lag Management:** Manage jet lag by adjusting your sleep-wake cycle gradually, staying hydrated, and exposing yourself to natural light during daylight hours to help regulate your body's internal clock.

5. Hydration and Nutrition:
  - **Stay Hydrated:** Drink plenty of water throughout your travels to stay hydrated, support digestion, and maintain overall well-being, especially in warm climates or during long flights.
  - **Pack Healthy Snacks:** Bring along nutritious snacks like nuts, seeds, fruits, or whole grain crackers to avoid unhealthy temptations and maintain energy levels between meals.

6. Cultural Immersion:
  - **Mindful Experiences:** Immerse yourself in the local culture by participating in mindful experiences such as cooking classes, cultural tours, or meditation sessions that deepen your connection to the destination and promote well-being.
  - **Engage with Nature:** Spend time outdoors in natural settings, whether it's visiting parks, beaches, or scenic landscapes, to rejuvenate your spirit and foster a sense of tranquility and connection with the environment.

7. Self-Care Practices:
  - **Daily Rituals:** Maintain your self-care routines while traveling, whether it's practicing yoga, journaling, or enjoying a cup of tea in the morning, to nurture your mental, emotional, and spiritual well-being.
  - **Set Boundaries:** Prioritize your well-being by setting boundaries and knowing when to say no to activities or commitments that may compromise your health or enjoyment during your travels.

8. Adaptability and Flexibility:
  - **Embrace Uncertainty:** Approach travel with an open mind and a sense of adventure, embracing the unexpected and viewing challenges as opportunities for growth and learning.
  - **Be Flexible:** Stay flexible with your plans and expectations, allowing room for spontaneity and serendipitous discoveries that enrich your travel experience and promote holistic well-being.

9. Connect with Locals:
  - **Cultural Exchange:** Engage in meaningful interactions with locals to learn about their traditions, customs, and way of life, fostering connections and expanding your cultural awareness and empathy.

- **Volunteer Opportunities:** Consider volunteering or participating in community-based initiatives that allow you to give back to the local community and contribute to positive social impact during your travels.

10. Reflection and Gratitude:
- **Journaling:** Keep a travel journal to reflect on your experiences, insights, and moments of gratitude, fostering self-awareness and appreciation for the richness of your journey.
- **Express Gratitude:** Practice gratitude daily by acknowledging and expressing gratitude for the people, experiences, and blessings you encounter during your travels, cultivating a positive mindset and deepening your sense of well-being.

Mind-Body-Spirit Approaches to Jet Lag

Managing jet lag holistically involves addressing the physical, mental, and spiritual aspects of well-being to minimize its effects and promote a smooth transition to a new time zone. Here are holistic mind-body-spirit approaches to managing jet lag:

1. Prepare Mindfully:
- **Sleep Adjustment:** Gradually adjust your sleep schedule a few days before your trip to align with your destination's time zone, helping your body adapt more smoothly to the new schedule.
- **Hydration:** Stay well-hydrated before, during, and after your flight to support physical well-being and counteract dehydration caused by air travel.

2. Mind-Body Techniques:
- **Mindful Breathing:** Practice deep breathing exercises or meditation during your flight to promote relaxation, reduce stress, and alleviate tension in the body.
- **Yoga and Stretching:** Incorporate gentle yoga poses or stretching exercises during long flights to improve circulation, relieve muscle stiffness, and enhance overall comfort.

3. Natural Remedies:

- **Herbal Supplements:** Consider natural remedies such as melatonin, valerian root, or chamomile tea to support sleep regulation and relaxation while adjusting to a new time zone.
- **Essential Oils:** Use calming essential oils like lavender or peppermint to create a soothing atmosphere and promote relaxation during your travels.

4. Light Exposure:

- **Natural Light:** Expose yourself to natural sunlight upon arrival at your destination to help reset your circadian rhythm and signal to your body that it's time to wake up and adjust to the local time.
- **Light Therapy:** Use light therapy devices or lamps to simulate natural daylight exposure, particularly in the morning, if adjusting to a new time zone during the winter or in locations with limited sunlight.

5. Grounding Practices:

- **Earthing:** Spend time outdoors barefoot, connecting with the earth's surface, to ground yourself and promote a sense of balance and vitality after long flights.
- **Nature Walks:** Take leisurely walks in natural settings like parks or gardens to reconnect with nature, reduce stress, and enhance overall well-being during your travels.

6. Cultural Immersion:

- **Local Rituals:** Embrace local customs or rituals related to sleep and relaxation in your destination, whether it's enjoying a traditional herbal tea before bed or participating in a mindfulness practice unique to the culture.
- **Cultural Activities:** Engage in cultural activities or experiences that foster a sense of connection and belonging, helping you adjust to the new environment and time zone more seamlessly.

7. Spiritual Practices:

- **Meditation:** Dedicate time for meditation or reflection upon arrival at your destination, grounding yourself in the present moment and fostering inner peace and clarity amidst the transition.
- **Prayer or Rituals:** Engage in spiritual practices such as prayer, chanting, or rituals that resonate with your beliefs and values, providing comfort and support during times of change and adjustment.

8. Self-Care Rituals:
  - **Restorative Activities:** Prioritize self-care activities such as hot baths, massage, or gentle self-massage techniques to relax your body, calm your mind, and promote restorative sleep.
  - **Nourishing Nutrition:** Choose nourishing foods that support your well-being and energy levels, opting for light, nutrient-rich meals and snacks to fuel your body while adjusting to a new time zone.

9. Connection and Community:
  - **Share Experiences:** Connect with fellow travelers or locals to share experiences, tips, and support, fostering a sense of camaraderie and mutual understanding during the adjustment period.
  - **Community Wellness Events:** Seek out community wellness events or gatherings, such as yoga classes or meditation workshops, where you can connect with like-minded individuals and cultivate a sense of belonging.

10. Gratitude and Reflection:
  - **Gratitude Practice:** Cultivate gratitude for the opportunity to travel and explore new places, expressing appreciation for the journey and experiences that lie ahead.
  - **Reflective Journaling:** Keep a travel journal to document your thoughts, feelings, and experiences as you adjust to a new time zone, reflecting on moments of growth, insight, and gratitude along the way.

Nurturing Well-Being in Different Cultures

Nurturing well-being while traveling in different cultures involves embracing the diversity of experiences and customs while prioritizing practices that promote holistic health. Here's how you can nurture well-being in different cultures:

1. Cultural Immersion:
  - **Open-mindedness:** Approach cultural differences with curiosity and respect, embracing new customs, traditions, and ways of life with an open mind and heart.

- **Cultural Awareness:** Educate yourself about the cultural norms, values, and etiquette of the places you visit to navigate interactions respectfully and authentically.

2. Mindful Eating:
- **Local Cuisine:** Explore the diverse flavors and ingredients of local cuisine, savoring traditional dishes that reflect the cultural heritage and culinary traditions of the region.
- **Mindful Eating Practices:** Practice mindful eating by paying attention to your senses, savoring each bite, and cultivating gratitude for the nourishment and cultural experience provided by the food.

3. Respectful Communication:
- **Language Learning:** Learn basic phrases and greetings in the local language to communicate respectfully and foster meaningful connections with locals.
- **Cultural Sensitivity:** Be mindful of cultural differences in communication styles, body language, and social customs, adapting your behavior accordingly to show respect and understanding.

4. Cultural Activities:
- **Local Traditions:** Participate in cultural activities and traditions such as festivals, ceremonies, or rituals that offer insights into the beliefs, values, and heritage of the community.
- **Art and Performance:** Attend local performances, art exhibits, or cultural demonstrations to immerse yourself in the creative expressions and artistic traditions of the culture.

5. Connection with Nature:
- **Natural Wonders:** Explore the natural beauty and landscapes of the region, whether it's hiking in mountains, swimming in oceans, or strolling through botanical gardens, to rejuvenate your spirit and connect with the environment.
- **Nature-Based Practices:** Engage in nature-based practices such as forest bathing, beach yoga, or sunset meditation to deepen your connection with nature and promote holistic well-being.

6. Community Engagement:

- **Local Communities:** Connect with local communities through volunteer opportunities, homestays, or cultural exchanges that offer authentic insights into daily life and foster meaningful relationships.

- **Support Local Businesses:** Patronize locally-owned businesses, markets, and artisans to support the local economy and contribute to sustainable tourism practices that benefit the community.

7. Mind-Body Practices:

- **Cultural Wellness Traditions:** Explore traditional wellness practices such as yoga, meditation, or traditional healing modalities that are integral to the culture's approach to holistic health and well-being.

- **Local Wellness Experiences:** Seek out local spas, hot springs, or wellness retreats that offer unique healing therapies and relaxation techniques rooted in the cultural heritage of the region.

8. Spiritual Exploration:

- **Sacred Sites:** Visit sacred sites, temples, or places of worship to learn about the spiritual beliefs and practices of the culture, honoring the sacredness of these spaces with reverence and mindfulness.

- **Personal Reflection:** Take time for personal reflection and introspection in sacred spaces or natural settings, connecting with your inner self and seeking inspiration from the cultural and spiritual richness of the environment.

9. Cross-Cultural Learning:

- **Cultural Exchange:** Engage in meaningful interactions with locals, exchanging stories, sharing meals, and learning from each other's perspectives to broaden your understanding and appreciation of different cultures.

- **Cultural Workshops:** Participate in cultural workshops or classes that teach traditional crafts, cooking techniques, or performing arts, allowing you to learn new skills and deepen your connection to the culture.

10. Gratitude and Respect:

- **Cultural Respect:** Show respect for local customs, traditions, and sacred sites by following cultural protocols, dressing modestly, and asking for permission before taking photographs.

- **Gratitude Practice:** Cultivate gratitude for the richness of cultural experiences, expressing appreciation for the hospitality, kindness, and wisdom shared by the people you encounter during your travels.

Creating Holistic Travel Plans

Creating holistic travel plans involves integrating mind, body, and spirit practices into your itinerary to prioritize well-being and enhance your travel experience. Here's how to create holistic travel plans:

1. **Set Intentions:**
 - **Reflective Practice:** Begin by reflecting on your travel goals and intentions, considering how you can align your trip with holistic principles that support mind-body wellness.
 - **Intentions Setting:** Set clear intentions for your journey, whether it's to relax, explore new cultures, or deepen your spiritual practice, guiding your decisions and activities throughout your travels.

2. **Mindful Destination Selection:**
 - **Research and Planning:** Conduct research on potential destinations, considering factors such as cultural offerings, outdoor activities, and wellness opportunities that resonate with your interests and values.
 - **Sustainable Travel:** Choose destinations that prioritize sustainability, environmental conservation, and responsible tourism practices to minimize your ecological footprint and support local communities.

3. **Holistic Accommodation Choices:**
 - **Wellness Retreats:** Consider staying at wellness resorts, eco-friendly lodges, or retreat centers that offer holistic amenities such as yoga classes, meditation sessions, spa treatments, and nutritious meals.
 - **Nature-Based Accommodation:** Opt for accommodations located in natural settings such as forests, mountains, or beaches, providing opportunities for outdoor activities and connection with nature.

4. **Mindful Packing:**

- **Essential Items:** Pack mindfully, including essential items such as comfortable clothing, sunscreen, insect repellent, reusable water bottles, and any medications or supplements you may need to support your well-being.
- **Mindful Consumption:** Pack light and conscientiously, minimizing waste and avoiding single-use plastics by bringing reusable bags, utensils, and containers for eco-friendly travel.

5. Balanced Itinerary:

- **Mind-Body-Spirit Activities:** Create a balanced itinerary that incorporates mind-body-spirit practices such as yoga, meditation, hiking, cultural excursions, and leisure time for relaxation and reflection.
- **Flexibility:** Allow for flexibility in your schedule to accommodate spontaneous experiences, unexpected opportunities, and moments of rest or self-care as needed.

6. Nutritious Eating:

- **Local Cuisine:** Explore local markets and restaurants to savor fresh, seasonal foods that nourish your body and provide insight into the culinary traditions of the region.
- **Healthy Snacks:** Pack nutritious snacks such as fruits, nuts, seeds, and whole grain crackers for sustenance during travel and between meals.

7. Movement and Exercise:

- **Outdoor Activities:** Plan outdoor activities such as hiking, cycling, swimming, or nature walks to engage in physical movement and connect with the natural beauty of your destination.
- **Mindful Movement:** Incorporate mindful movement practices such as yoga, tai chi, or qigong into your daily routine to promote flexibility, strength, and relaxation.

8. Cultural Immersion:

- **Local Experiences:** Immerse yourself in the local culture by participating in cultural activities, attending festivals, visiting historical sites, and interacting with locals to gain a deeper understanding of the destination.

- **Language Learning:** Learn basic phrases and greetings in the local language to facilitate communication and foster connections with the people you encounter during your travels.

9. Rest and Relaxation:
- **Downtime:** Schedule downtime for rest and relaxation, allowing yourself to unwind, recharge, and rejuvenate after busy days of exploration and activity.
- **Self-Care Rituals:** Practice self-care rituals such as journaling, reading, taking leisurely baths, or enjoying quiet moments of reflection to nurture your mental and emotional well-being.

10. Gratitude and Mindfulness:
- **Gratitude Practice:** Cultivate gratitude for the opportunities, experiences, and connections encountered during your travels, expressing appreciation for the beauty and abundance of the world around you.
- **Mindful Presence:** Practice mindfulness throughout your journey, savoring each moment with awareness and presence, whether it's admiring a breathtaking view, enjoying a delicious meal, or connecting with fellow travelers.

Sustainable and Mindful Tourism

Sustainable and mindful tourism involves traveling with respect for the environment, local communities, and cultural heritage while prioritizing personal well-being and holistic principles. Here's how to practice sustainable and mindful tourism:

1. Choose Sustainable Accommodations:
- **Eco-Friendly Lodges:** Opt for accommodations that prioritize sustainability practices such as energy efficiency, waste reduction, water conservation, and use of renewable resources.
- **Green Certifications:** Look for eco-certifications or sustainability labels that indicate a commitment to environmental stewardship and responsible tourism practices.

2. Reduce Environmental Impact:

   - **Minimize Waste:** Bring reusable water bottles, bags, and utensils to minimize single-use plastics and reduce waste during your travels.
   - **Conserve Resources:** Practice water and energy conservation in accommodations by limiting shower time, turning off lights and air conditioning when not in use, and reusing towels and linens.

 3. Support Local Communities:
   - **Buy Local:** Purchase goods and souvenirs from local artisans, markets, and cooperatives to support the local economy and promote cultural preservation.
   - **Responsible Dining:** Eat at locally-owned restaurants and street food stalls that source ingredients from local producers, reducing carbon emissions associated with food transportation and supporting small-scale agriculture.

 4. Respect Cultural Heritage:
   - **Cultural Sensitivity:** Respect local customs, traditions, and sacred sites by dressing modestly, following cultural etiquette, and seeking permission before taking photographs.
   - **Learn About Culture:** Educate yourself about the history, customs, and beliefs of the places you visit, fostering understanding and appreciation for the cultural heritage of the destination.

 5. Practice Mindful Travel:
   - **Slow Travel:** Embrace a slower pace of travel to immerse yourself in the local culture, connect with the community, and reduce your carbon footprint by minimizing air travel and opting for overland transportation.
   - **Mindful Consumption:** Be mindful of your consumption habits, opting for experiences over material possessions and choosing activities that align with your values and interests.

 6. Responsible Wildlife Encounters:
   - **Ethical Tours:** Choose wildlife tours and experiences that prioritize animal welfare, conservation, and responsible interaction with wildlife, avoiding activities that exploit or harm animals for entertainment.
   - **Respect Wildlife:** Observe wildlife from a safe distance, refrain from feeding or touching wild animals, and follow guidelines provided

by local authorities or tour operators to minimize disturbance to their natural habitat.

7. Support Sustainable Tourism Initiatives:

- **Volunteer Programs:** Participate in responsible volunteer programs or community-based tourism initiatives that contribute positively to local development, conservation efforts, and social welfare projects.
- **Conservation Projects:** Support conservation organizations and initiatives that work to protect natural habitats, wildlife, and cultural heritage sites through donations, volunteer work, or advocacy efforts.

8. Leave No Trace:

- **Pack Out What You Pack In:** Practice Leave No Trace principles by carrying out all waste and disposing of it properly, leaving natural areas and cultural sites as you found them.
- **Respect Nature:** Avoid damaging or disturbing natural ecosystems, plants, and wildlife by staying on designated trails, respecting wildlife habitats, and avoiding activities that cause harm to the environment.

9. Educate and Advocate:

- **Raise Awareness:** Share your experiences and knowledge about sustainable and mindful tourism with friends, family, and fellow travelers, inspiring others to make conscious choices and support responsible travel practices.
- **Advocate for Change:** Support policies and initiatives that promote sustainable tourism, environmental protection, and social justice, advocating for responsible tourism practices at local, national, and international levels.

10. Practice Gratitude and Mindfulness:

- **Gratitude Practice:** Cultivate gratitude for the beauty and diversity of the natural world, the hospitality of local communities, and the transformative experiences encountered during your travels.
- **Mindful Presence:** Practice mindfulness throughout your journey, savoring each moment with awareness and appreciation, whether it's witnessing a stunning sunset, tasting a delicious local dish, or connecting with the local culture.